Why Exercise?

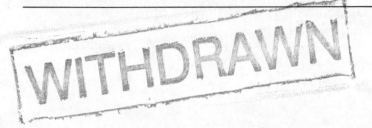

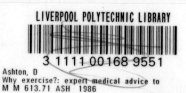

This book is dedicated to all those who would like to assume a greater degree of responsibility for their own health.

Why Exercise?

*Expert medical advice to help you enjoy
a healthier life*

David Ashton and Bruce Davies
With cartoons by Larry

Basil Blackwell

Copyright © David Ashton and Bruce Davies 1986

First published 1986

Basil Blackwell Ltd
108 Cowley Road, Oxford OX4 1JF, UK

Basil Blackwell Inc.
432 Park Avenue South, Suite 1503,
New York, NY 10016, USA

British Library Cataloguing in Publication Data
Ashton, David
  Why exercise?
  1. Exercise
  I. Title   II. Davies, Bruce
  613.7'1   RA787

  ISBN 0-631-14174-X
  ISBN 0-631-14175-8 Pbk

Library of Congress Cataloging in Publication Data
Ashton, David
  Why exercise?

  Bibliography: p.
  Includes index.
  1. Exercise. 2. Heart—Diseases—Prevention—Popular
works. I. Davies, Bruce. II. Title. [DNLM:
1. Exertion—popular works. 2. Physical Fitness—
popular works. QT 255 A828y]
RA781.A76 1986   613.7   86-12919
ISBN 0-631-14174-X
ISBN 0-631-14175-8 (pbk.)

Typeset in 10/12pt Plantin by
Katerprint Typesetting Services, Oxford
Printed in Great Britain by Page Bros (Norwich) Ltd

Contents

About the Authors

Dr David Ashton

Dr David Ashton qualified in medicine at the University of St Andrews and Victoria University of Manchester; having gained several academic distinctions, he went on to pursue post-graduate training. At present he is Medical Director for American Medical International and is also a member of the University Department of Cardiology at Manchester Royal Infirmary.

David Ashton has a particular interest in the primary prevention of cardiovascular disease but is also committed to the whole spectrum of preventive medicine. He is currently engaged in a number of areas of research and has special experience in the clinical applications of exercise stress testing; post-coronary rehabilitation; the relationship between exercise and coronary heart disease and the prevention of sudden cardiac death. He has been Medical Adviser to several world-class athletes and in this context is especially interested in the effects of viral illness on athletic performance. David Ashton has vast experience of cardiovascular assessment and exercise prescription in a wide spectrum of individuals, including those with established cardiovascular disease.

Dr Bruce Davies

Dr Bruce Davies is Senior Lecturer in Physiology in the Department of Biological Sciences at the University of Salford. He is at present on a three-year secondment to American Medical International as the Technical Director of their programme for preventive medicine. For the past nine years he has been the Technical Director of the Preston Post-coronary Rehabilitation Programme and in this capacity he has supervised more than 60,000 man hours of post-coronary exercise. Bruce Davies has a special interest in the clinical applications of exercise stress testing and has supervised more than 10,000 such investigations. He has published numerous scientific papers in edited journals and has addressed many international conferences. He is a Fellow of the American College of Sports Medicine and has gained an international reputation for his work in preventive medicine and post-coronary rehabilitation. He is also an honorary Research Fellow at the Department of Medicine in Preston Royal Infirmary. Dr Davies has been the Physiological Adviser to six Olympic teams and is currently the consulting physiologist to the senior Welsh National rugby squad.

Bruce Davies's work has embraced the whole spectrum of human activity from the exercising spina bifida child and paraplegic to the world's fastest marathon runner. He is a frequent broadcaster and has made numerous television and radio appearances. He is, without question, one of Britain's leading authorities on the clinical prescription and application of exercise.

Foreword

It is my hope that the readers of this book will find that the knowledge contained within it will be of practical value in their quest for health and fitness. Athletics offers a challenging area for scientific and medical research. However, exercise should not be the province of an elite few who strive for the highest levels of athletic performance. The most remarkable property of exercise is its power to promote and maintain health and it is this aspect to which we should now be addressing ourselves.

I have always found it extremely stimulating and rewarding to work with the authors. Not only is the knowledge of their results helpful in my own pursuit of excellence; I am sure they will ultimately be of great value to all individuals who wish to pursue a healthier and more active life style.

Steve Jones
Marathon Runner

Preface

As ever more runners appear on our streets and those few film stars and television personalities who have not yet produced a book on health and fitness settle down to work, now is perhaps a good time to consider whether the current increase in leisure-time exercise is really doing us any good. Many of those in the vanguard of the present fitness movement or 'leisure industry' as it is now called, have been motivated less by any truly altruistic intentions of improving the health of the population, than by the promise of considerable commercial and financial success. When the present wave of enthusiasm for 'aerobics' and other forms of exercise has passed, the entrepreneurs will await the arrival of the next potentially lucrative fashion.

To date an extraordinary number of books on exercise and health have been produced and, since commercial success demands at least some claim to originality, each 'expert' or showbusiness personality has invented an apparently unique formula for health, beauty, fitness and even success. The reasoning behind books of this kind is not difficult to discern: if you buy the particular book written by X, and dutifully perform what X recommends, you will eventually end up looking like X. The reality of course is somewhat less spectacular, but that has not deterred thousands of 'hopefuls' from joining their local health club or fitness studio.

These developments have had a number of important and sometimes undesirable effects. First, many people who would be prepared to become involved in exercise are dissuaded from doing so because they do not think of themselves as possessors of the slim, svelte, sun-tanned bodies so beloved of the advertising industry and image-makers. Consequently they may feel embarrassed at the prospect of turning up at their local health club, or running on the roads, for fear that they would look ridiculous. Few of us have the physique or looks of the models who advertise sportswear, nor is it particularly desirable that we should. Nevertheless, the current obsession with personal appearance and the 'cosmetic' effects of exercise has diverted attention away from the far more important issue, which is the relationship between exercise, health and disease. Whilst it is true that many people who take exercise are vaguely aware that it may be doing them some good, experience suggests that they are poorly informed as to *why* regular exercise may be beneficial.

Secondly, there has been so much nonsense and 'dis-information' written about exercise in recent years, that lay people and health professionals alike have become confused about the possible benefits and risks of advising increased activity. This situation has been compounded by the mass of pseudo-scientific jargon which now pervades the exercise movement and which lends the 'experts' an aura of quite unjustified scientific credibility. The popular press and other media have done little to dispel the confusion. There has been a tendency to trivialize the issues; anyone involved in regular exercise and who takes more than a passing interest in his/her own health runs the risk of being labelled a 'fitness fanatic'.

The newspapers also have a penchant for reporting the more tragic features of exercise. Heart attacks and even cases of sudden death which can be shown to have some connection with exercise, however tenuous, are seized upon with a morbid sensationalism. The lay public, understandably, has a tendency to perceive this as clear evidence that exercise is harmful, and biased journalism of this kind serves only to obscure the real issue still further.

It is estimated that there are as many as two million regular 'joggers' in the United Kingdom. We have yet to see a newspaper headline proclaiming that 'Two Million Take Exercise This Week With No Casualties'. It does not, after all, make exciting news. On the day when Jim Fixx, a leader of the American fitness movement, died suddenly whilst running in America, many thousands more died partly as a consequence of *not* exercising regularly. The potential benefits of regular exercise far outweigh any potential dangers, and the risk of not exercising is very much greater. In the midst of all the controversy and confusion and press exaggeration it comes as no surprise that many people simply sit back in their armchairs and hope the whole thing will go away.

In this book we have argued for the simple proposition that much of our present disease burden is preventable and that exercise has a powerful role to play in both preventing disease and promoting health. The role of exercise should not be considered in isolation, however, and many other factors, which are no less important, must also be taken into account. By considering the role of exercise within the framework of an overall health strategy, we hope that the reader will understand both its importance and its limitations.

Attitudes towards health in this country are slow to change and if we are to encourage more people to become physically active and to assume a greater degree of responsibility for their own health then every effort must be made to provide clear and concise advice, which is based upon scientific evidence rather than hearsay. This book is an attempt to do just that, and we hope that the reader will be encouraged to pursue a healthier and more active lifestyle.

This book does not contain all the answers. We gladly accept in advance any criticism for its many imperfections.

W.D.A.
B.D.

Acknowledgements

We would like to thank Terry Thomas, Bob Mathers and Malcolm Hurlston for reading the manuscript and providing constructive criticism. We would also like to thank Professor Reg Beech at the Department of Clinical Psychology, University of South Manchester, for his help and advice concerning the assessment of personality and its relationship to stress. Thanks also to Dr Derek Rowlands, Consultant Cardiologist at Manchester Royal Infirmary, and Dr Douglas Watt, Consultant Physician at the Royal Preston Hospital, for their skill and guidance in the management of many of our more difficult patients. Special thanks are due to Alison Oldham for her skill and enthusiasm in the typing and preparation of the manuscript. We would also like to thank Blackwells for managing to turn a rather large and unwieldy original manuscript into a balanced and well ordered book.

Finally, we would like to thank Steve Jones, probably the greatest marathon runner in the world. His awesome commitment to his own search for excellence continues to be a source of inspiration and encouragement to us all.

1

Physical Activity in Man – the Element of Choice

> If some of the benefits accruing from regular exercise could be procured by any one Medicine, then nothing in the World would be held in more esteem than that Medicine.
>
> *Francis Fuller*

Francis Fuller was a man ahead of his time. In 1705 he published a remarkable book called *Medicina-Gymnastica*, or to give its full and more descriptive title, 'A Treatise on the Power of Exercise with respect to the Animal Economy, and the Great Necessity of it in the cure of Several Distempers'. Although Fuller himself died less than 12 months later, at the age of only 36, his book continued to be published for many years after his death. The ninth edition, the last, was produced in 1777.

Leafing through the pages of his book today, one cannot fail to be impressed by Fuller's remarkable insight into the relationship between physical activity and health, all the more extraordinary, since he would have been almost entirely ignorant of the complex physiological and biochemical mechanisms by which the benefits of exercise are achieved.

From the health and disease point of view, our own period of history differs from that of Fuller in two important respects. First, the major causes of disability and death (morbidity and mortality) in the seventeenth and eighteenth centuries were the infectious diseases, such as smallpox, diphtheria, typhoid, dysentery and tuberculosis. The last recorded case of plague in England was in 1669, although there had been a dreadful epidemic in 1665.

The twentieth century epidemics are rather different. They have been called the diseases of 'civilization', since they are generally rare in Third World and developing countries. Coronary heart disease and cancer are the major causes of premature disability and death in our own society, and deaths from infections are rare in comparison. Another important point to note is that to a large extent the burden of disease which Western society suffers at present is self-inflicted. If we choose to smoke cigarettes and run the risk of lung cancer or heart disease, then we are doing so in the full knowledge of the possible consequences of our actions. Those who died from infectious diseases in Fuller's time were unable to exercise any control or rational choice concerning their health. This is the paradox of twentieth century man; he has the means at his disposal to provide a level of health and well-being for the population unheard of in previous generations yet he has failed to do so.

The second major difference between Francis Fuller's time and our own is the extensive development of science and technology and its influence on our understanding of the mechanisms and complexities of the human organism. That is not to imply that we have all the answers – far from it – but we do have a level of understanding of health and disease that is vastly beyond anything available to Fuller. The basic principles of physiology, biochemistry and psychology have been enunciated, and since the turn of the century there has been what can only be described as an 'explosion' of knowledge in medicine and science. In the past 30 years or so, scientists have increasingly addressed themselves to the possible relationship between activity patterns and health, providing a new and exciting dimension of research. The irony is that, despite this torrent of information, modern day scientists' conclusions are much the same as those Fuller reached all those years ago. The essential difference, of course, is that we now have the scientific understanding he lacked, although whether this makes any practical difference is arguable.

This book will discuss the evidence relating physical activity patterns to health and disease. We do not ignore the other important factors, such as diet, smoking, obesity etc., nor are we suggesting that physical activity is necessarily the most important of the many influences on our health and well-being. We do believe, however, that exercise can and does have profound effects upon the body and mind, and that hitherto its power as a means of disease prevention, rehabilitation and health enhancement has been very largely neglected by orthodox medical practice.

During the past decade or so we have witnessed a tremendous increase in interest and participation in many forms of leisure-time activity. This phenomenon is vividly illustrated by the current mass participation in marathon running and 'aerobics', both of which have already achieved huge followings in the USA. Marathon running in particular seems to have caught the public imagination, and many thousands of hitherto sedentary, middle-aged individuals are donning their tracksuits and running shorts, intent on completing the mystical 26 miles 385 yards. So great has the current interest become that we are quite accustomed to hearing about the 'fitness boom' or the 'leisure industry'.

There are many reasons for this extraordinary change in attitude, but two main factors seem to be paramount. First, the increased availability of leisure time means that many individuals now have the opportunity to develop a sporting interest. Secondly, more and more people are realizing that exercise may be of some benefit in terms of health, although the evidence would suggest that they are very poorly informed as to exactly how. Participation in mass exercise is a twentieth century phenomenon, at least in Britain. To understand its emergence during the past decade or so, it is necessary to examine the role of physical activity in the evolution of man, and the development of our modern concept of leisure time.

Leisure – an Evolving Concept

Primitive Man

Ancient man evolved as a 'hunter–gatherer'. In other words his metabolism* was designed to allow a physically active mode of existence and to obtain nutrition and sustenance from a mainly vegetarian diet. For virtually all of the four million years that man has walked this planet he has lived mainly on plants, berries, fruit and other vegetables, with animal sources of proteins such as meat and fish as a supplement to his diet. Hunting animals required a certain degree of social organization, together with the necessary weapons, and life was dangerous. The popular idea of the hairy caveman, club in hand, dragging the carcass of some enormous animal back to his cave is wildy inaccurate.

It is true that man is, strictly speaking, an omnivore, that is, he is able to derive energy from a very wide range of food sources, both animal and vegetable. Nevertheless, the correct emphasis should be placed upon the gathering rather than the hunting, the vegetable rather than the animal. The important point, however, is that both hunting and gathering demanded a certain level of physical activity. Indeed, man's survival depended so much on his remaining mobile that a broken limb could well have had catastrophic consequences. Exercise was not, therefore, a question of choice, but a *sine qua non* of remaining alive.

In terms of man's basic diet, and the extent to which physical activity remained an integral part of his everyday existence, little changed until very recent times. What changes did occur were gradual, allowing a normal process of adaptation of man to his environment. As societies grew and flourished, methods of growing crops and other vegetable sources of

---

* For definitions of this and other terms used in this book, please see the glossary on pp. 233–6.

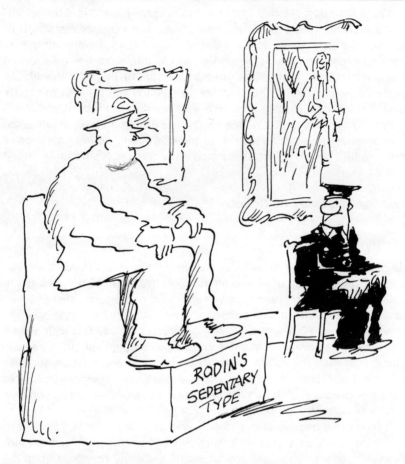

food were introduced, constituting a primitive form of agriculture. The vast majority of the population were land workers, and this has remained so for virtually the whole of human history. Even as recently as 1900, approximately 60 per cent of the American population lived on farms.

Tilling the soil, planting and harvesting the various crops, cutting wood, all involved lifting, pushing, carrying, walking and other forms of exertion. Life was thus physically extremely hard, and little free time was generally available for relaxation or recreation. Nevertheless, the lot of the farmworker was probably better than the miserable existence of the increasing numbers of people who sought work in the towns and the cities.

1700–1900: the Industrial Revolution

The period from 1700 to 1900 marked a profound change in man's evolution. Major changes in the economic life of the country must necessarily disturb the whole social structure, and in this respect the industrial revolution was no exception. Indeed, the environmental and social conditions for vast numbers of people were to change more radically than at any other time in history. Although this was to be the period during which science and technology would revolutionize agriculture and industry, the initial changes were not strictly of a technological nature. Despite the high mortality from infectious diseases, the population of Britain increased substantially from 1700 onwards. This was due mainly to improved methods of food production as a result of the agricultural revolution, which had spread throughout Europe from the seventeenth century onwards.

From about 1800, the industrial revolution, with its increased mechanization and organization, began to take a firmer hold. Compared with the centuries that had gone before, the changes in industry, agriculture and social life of the second half of the eighteenth century were both violent and revolutionary. The new factories required labour, and a mass migration of workers from the country into the towns and cities began. Rural poverty and the fear of the workhouse was the motivating factor in most cases – indeed the towns and cities offered the only real hope of wages and food for many people.

Working conditions were often appalling. Factories were built without any regard for the welfare or health of the individuals who were to labour in them. The workers were exploited ruthlessly and accidents and occupational diseases were commonplace. Compensation was unheard of. In the early part of the century only about one child in four born in London survived, and the infant mortality rate was probably even higher in the towns and cities of the Midlands and the North.

Physical activity was as integral a part of everyday life as ever before, but now it was directed towards different ends. Farm workers had physically arduous lives, but they at least had the benefit of open air and sunshine. Factory workers spent long hours in filthy, noisy and dimly lit workshops, with little opportunity to enjoy the countryside. They worked long hours for low wages and female and child labour was exploited to the full. Life in the mines and the cotton mills was barely tolerable, but the domestic circumstances were no better. Friedrich Engels provides a vivid description of the living conditions of the cotton mill workers of Manchester, the 'shock-City of the 1850s':

Masses of refuse, offal, and sickening filth lie among standing pools in all directions; the atmosphere is poisoned by the effluvia from these, and laden and darkened by the smoke of a dozen tall factory chimneys. A hoard of ragged women and children swarm about here as filthy as the swine that thrive upon the garbage heaps and in the puddles . . .

The race that lives in these ruinous cottages, behind broken windows, mended with oilskins, sprung doors, and rotten doorposts, or in dark, wet cellars, in measureless filth and stench, in this atmosphere penned in as if with a purpose, this race must really have reached the lowest stage of humanity.

Not surprisingly the major cause of death was infectious disease of one form or another, but particularly typhoid, diphtheria and dysentery. The children who worked in the cotton mills or the coalmines had neither the time nor the strength to play. For them and their parents life was simply a succession of working days, and whatever free time was available was spent in recovering from the day's toil. The concept of 'leisure' time, as we understand the term, would have been meaningless to them. Physical activity in the form of the endless drudgery of the mill, or the back-breaking toil of the mines, was an all too prominent feature of their existence. The danger for these people was not that they could not take sufficient exercise, but that they were in danger of literally working themselves to death.

The Twentieth Century

The twentieth century heralded the technological revolution, which was to have even greater social and environmental consequences than the industrial revolution which preceded it. During the past 40 years in particular, we have witnessed a quite staggering increase in scientific and technological expertise, which has left scarcely any part of our lives untouched. Space technology has allowed man to begin the exploration of our solar system, and computers have become part and parcel of our everyday life. Indeed, it is our proud boast that we are able to manufacture cars 'untouched by human hands'. If Arkwright's Water Frame (1769) and Hargreaves' Jenny (1770) were the symbols of the industrial revolution, then data banks, word processors and laser communication systems have become the symbols of the new technology.

There are three main areas in which the application of technological expertise at the most sophisticated level has had enormous consequences for our environment and our lifestyle.

Agriculture and food production

The Western diet has changed enormously during the past 100 years. We now consume vast amounts of meat and other animal produce, and far less in the way of vegetable sources of nutrition, than at any other time in our history. Our intake of animal fat, sugar and salt has increased to unprecedented levels. Figures 1.1 and 1.2 illustrate how the intake of fats, meat

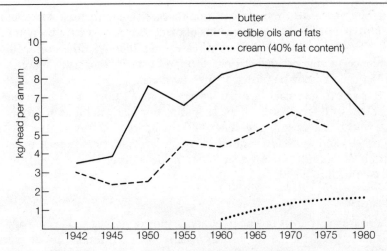

Figure 1.1   Fat intake per head per annum since the end of the Second World War.

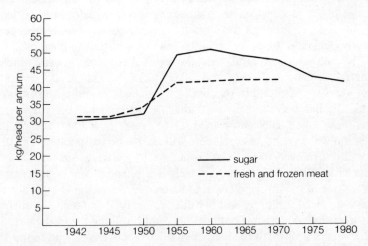

Figure 1.2   Intake of sugar and meat per head per annum since the end of the Second World War.

and sugar per head, per annum has increased very substantially since the Second World War.

We now know that this change in our diet has had appalling consequences and numerous reports[*] in recent years have recommended that we should substantially reduce our intake of animal fats, sugar and salt.

---

[*] The National Advisory Committee on Nutrition, Education (NACNE) 1983; The Committee on Medical Aspects of Food Policy (COMA), 1984.

There is also a clear recommendation that we should increase the amount of fibre in our diets. Large amounts of dietary animal fat have been linked very closely to coronary heart disease, and there is other compelling evidence to suggest that various forms of cancer, especially bowel and breast cancer, may be related to high fat diets.

It is an extraordinary fact that for most of man's time on earth the major problem with food has been the lack of it. For many millions of people in the world that is still true. For Western nations, however, there is no shortage, and substantial numbers of us are suffering from a massive surfeit of calories. Obesity, in Western 'developed' countries, is now a major threat to health.

Medicine

There are many areas in which the application of science and technology in medicine has achieved spectacular success. Modern techniques of anaesthesia permit surgical procedures of enormous complexity. Organ transplatation, particularly cardiac and kidney transplants, attract extensive coverage in the media. Genetic engineering is now a reality, rather than a plausible theory, although the morality and the ethics of such procedures are hotly debated. We now live in the era of sophisticated diagnostic aids such as computerized axial tomography (CAT scanning) and nuclear magnetic resonance. These, and other technological developments in recent years, have added to our swelling armamentarium against disease. The public has become convinced that no matter what the ailment, no matter how much they abuse themselves or for how long, the medical profession will have an answer; there will always be an operation or a drug that will return everything to its normal healthy state again.

The pharmaceutical industry, which is a phenomenon of the past 40 years, is one of the most powerful industrial forces in the world. With its massive financial resources and bewildering array of drugs and medicines, it has managed to convince both the lay public and the medical profession itself that the answer to modern epidemics of disease can be found in a prescription. It is true that modern medicine has made many useful and life-saving contributions to health care, but we have a national drug problem in Britain which has assumed gargantuan proportions. The peoples of the developed world have become drug-takers and television watchers, content to sit back and let medicines solve their problems. For example, it is estimated that 40–50 per cent of American women will use tranquillizers at some point in their lives.

We have been seduced by the idea that high technology medicine will provide the answer, when there is in fact overwhelming evidence to the contrary. It is a matter of fact that most of the major reductions in mortality that have occurred during the past 200 years or so owed little to medical science. We have already seen that the major cause of death in the past was infectious diseases. These were dealt with not by the contributions of medical science, but rather by the advent of improved living conditions and nutrition. The substantial reduction in death rates which occurred during the eighteenth and nineteenth century pre-dates by a long way the introduction of antibiotics in the 1930s.

Concerning the modern epidemics of heart disease and cancer, the emphasis has hitherto been directed towards treatment of the established condition, rather than prevention. Massive resources are directed towards the development of drugs and surgery for the treatment of coronary heart disease, to the detriment of research into methods of prevention. We have substantial evidence to suggest that simple changes in diet and patterns of physical activity could make a major contribution to the health and well-being of the population of this country. Yet the profession itself has failed to provide any real lead in this direction. The myth of the omnipotent medical profession remains, and is still unquestioningly accepted by most people. Even some doctors themselves have come to believe it.

These ideas have mitigated against the individual assuming responsibility for his or her own health and have created a tremendous dependence upon doctors, which many of them have encouraged. In most cases this was probably not intentional, but the result is that many people are addicted to their family doctor, to the point where almost every minor ailment, any slight deviation from what they perceive as the norm, requires a visit to the doctor and the almost inevitable prescription. Medical dependency is not good for your health, and an unquestioning belief in its power to heal may easily detract attention from the factors creating the illness in the first place.

The domestic and working environment

The impact of science and technology in the home and working environment has been as great as that in medicine and agriculture. Since the turn of this century we have witnessed the transformation of a physically active and essentially rural society into a population of town and city dwellers whose lifestyles have changed dramatically from that of their forefathers. Modern technology has now made it possible for us to live comfortably with the absolute minimum of physical effort. The development of the motor car is the most obvious example of such change, but there are countless other areas in which technology has left its mark.

Lifts and escalators relieve us of the need to negotiate the stairs in our offices and department stores. The effort of mowing the lawn at home has been greatly reduced since the advent of the power mower, and some have even opted for artificial grass! We can now play golf without necessarily having to walk between shots. In the home dishwashers and all sorts of other 'labour-saving' devices have appeared, and we can even change the channel on the television set without rising from the chair. Many people in this country and the USA will spend up to six hours a day watching television. This approximates (assuming a lifespan of three score years and ten), to 16 or 17 years across the average lifetime. This progessive application of technology to our daily lives will continue for the foreseeable future, and during the next decade or so it is likely that we shall be able to order the weekly shopping without even going to the supermarket. The paradox, of course, is that our soft and obese bodies are crying out for more physical activity, and yet we are engaged in the business of ensuring that they have to perform less and less.

In particular the application of technology to our working and domestic environments has given us an amount of leisure time which is without parallel in the whole of man's history: it is a twentieth century phenomenon.

A Fatal Combination

The process we have examined, in which the rise of industrialization and technology has exerted an enormous impact on our lives, has produced a number of serious risk factors to our health. The application of technology in food production and industry has helped to produce a diet high in animal fat (including cholesterol), processed sugar and salt, and the changes in our home and working environments have meant that we have become a highly sedentary population. These trends, in turn, are associated with an over-reliance on medicine and an unrealistic expectation of its power to heal. The present disease epidemics in Western society – coronary heart disease, hypertension, obesity, constipation, backache, cancer, depression and many other problems – are a reflection of our present lifestyles. They will not go away of their own accord. It is no use hoping that someone will produce a magic drug or surgical procedure that will lift this burden. Prevention is the best possible area for our attention from this point onwards.

You may ask why the factors we have mentioned should be reflected in such a high death rate from heart disease, and cancer and other ailments. After all, many people prefer to sit in front of the television, smoking and drinking. Many of us like to have cream teas and sweets and take the minimum of physical activity. Why should all these things mean that we are risking our lives? The answer is that living organisms can adapt to changes in their environment *provided that the changes occur gradually*, and that those better equipped to survive, from a genetic point of view, will continue to reproduce. The changes in human lifestyle and environment that we have discussed have occurred mainly during the past 100 years, and in evolutionary terms this insult to our metabolism is *instantaneous*. From being a highly active 'hunter–gatherer', man has overnight become 'homo sedentarius'. Millions of years of evolutionary adaptation allowed us to live in harmony with our environment until the advent of technology this century. We have been suddenly pitched into a modern, high-technology environment with its high speed and sophistication, but our bodies are metabolically alienated, unable to cope with the sudden onslaught.

It is quite possible that if the changes we have discussed had occurred over a sufficient period of time, adaptations would have occurred, and by a process of selection we could have developed the necessary metabolism to cope with the changes. But human reproduction is slow, and no such adaptation has occurred. Man, from a scientific and technological point of view, has entered a 'New World', but he is physiologically and metabolically tied to the old. The changes in diet, environment and activity patterns which we have discussed have been profound, but it is the *rapidity* with which these changes have occurred, allowing no time for adaptation, which has been the major factor in the development of the modern disease epidemics.

The Way Ahead

Medicine in this country has hitherto concerned itself primarily with diagnosing and treating established disease. Many distinguished scientists and physicians believe that in doing so it has made a fundamental error. They believe there is an urgent need to re-think the premises upon which the practice of orthodox medicine is based. Much greater resources and efforts must now be directed towards disease prevention and the enhancement of health, rather than the more negative approach which is so prevalent. Medicine needs to go on the *offensive* and become much more positive in its approach. Good health is not simply the absence of disease, it also has a much more positive dimension.

We have examined a number of risk factors that have been shown to be of great importance in the development of twentieth century diseases. In our view, one of the most important is the lack of physical activity. We have indicated that the concept of leisure time is a modern one; since physical exertion was such an integral part of everyday life until the present century, it has never been necessary to consider it as a separate entity. Our modern day lack of physical exertion, and the large amount of leisure time now available, now make it necessary to decide whether we shall use some of that time for physical exercise. In other words, from being a necessity, physical exercise is now a choice. Most of us choose to avoid it. Yet there are signs that increasing numbers of people are recognizing that health is their own responsibility, and that regular moderate exercise can do much to preserve well-being and provide an excellent quality of life.

We shall see later that there is substantial evidence to suggest that leisure-time exercise can make a major contribution to health. In our view, regular programmes of moderate exercise are the cornerstone of good health policy. This is because exercise has beneficial effects on most of the other risk factors. We believe also that it has a major part to play in disease prevention and in health enhancement. That is not to say that it is the panacea for all our health problems, but we could not do better than make it a foundation for future action.

We began this chapter with a discussion of a late seventeenth century writer, and it seems appropriate to end with some lines from another writer of the period, the English Poet Laureate, John Dryden. He summarizes elegantly and succinctly what we have attempted to say thus far:

> The wise, for cure, on exercise depend,
> God never made His work for Man to mend.

2

Heart Disease in the 1980s

Coronary heart disease is perhaps the most devastating epidemic ever to afflict Western society. In the United Kingdom alone it is responsible for about 150,000 deaths per year – one person every three to four minutes. One man in 11 can now expect to die of a heart attack before he is 65 years old, and for males between the ages of 45 to 64 years, more than two out of every five deaths are the consequence of coronary heart disease. Despite the improvements observed in the United States of America during the past decade, coronary heart disease there still acounts for more than half a million deaths each year, the figure in 1982 being 552,786.

The immediate mortality of a heart attack is approximately 40 per cent and of those who die, 25 per cent will do so instantaneously or within the first 15 minutes. Indeed, sudden death may be the first and only manifestation of a disease which kills indiscriminately and which is no respecter of age, position or social class. The cost in economic terms is enormous but the human cost is incalculable. Indeed, so prevalent has this disease become, that few of us cannot think of a relative, a friend or acquaintance who has not fallen one of its victims.

Strangely, familiarity in this case has bred not so much contempt, as apathy. There is a terrible sense of inevitability and defeatism among the medical profession and the general public alike and people seem resigned to accepting this appalling annual loss of life as part of everyday experience. We have lost our sense of indignation and outrage. This attitude, born of both fear and ignorance, is not, however, an appropriate response. The problem should not be accepted – it should be attacked. In those countries such as the USA where the problem is taken seriously there has, during the past decade or so, been a marked reduction in death rates from coronary heart disease. Unfortunately, successive governments in this country have failed to address this problem with any sense of urgency, which has mitigated against the formation of a rational, coordinated and concerted effort to deal with the problem. As a result, the lay public is still poorly informed about the factors responsible for the present epidemic, and many people still believe that heart disease is a normal and perhaps even necessary accompaniment to old age. To some extent this is true, but it ignores the fact that many thousands of young people are killed or prematurely disabled by a disease that no longer confines its interests to those who are 70 and over. The *average* age of patients on our own coronary rehabilitation programme is 45, and we have several patients who are still in their twenties.

Coronary heart disease is another twentieth century phenomenon. When Francis Fuller was writing about the benefits of exercise at the beginning of the eighteenth century the disease would have been unheard of and it was not until 1772 that the first clinical description of the heart condition, angina pectoris, was provided by the English physician William Heberden. Perhaps even more remarkable, however, is that as recently as the 1920s and 1930s, coronary heart disease was still regarded as an uncommon disease. Conversations with older colleagues who were practising medicine at that time certainly confirms it, and in his classic textbook of medicine the great physician Sir William Osler wrote in 1920: 'Angina Pectoris is a rare disease in hospitals, a case a year is about the average, even in the large metropolitan hospitals.' In the 1940s the disease became more common and accounted for approximately 20,000 deaths per year. By 1983, however, the figure was almost 160,000, and the disease is now by far the commonest cause of death.

Man's technological genius has created an environment which, for many, has become incompatible with survival. In this chapter and the next we shall be discussing the nature of coronary heart disease and examining those factors which are known to be of importance in its causation.

First, some discussion of simple anatomy and an explanation of the more common terminology is required.

The Heart of the Matter

Since antiquity, the heart has occupied a powerful position in the emotions of human beings, presumably because there is a readily apparent association between respiration, which depends upon the heart, and continued existence. The central part which the heart plays in our imagination, both individually and collectively, is illustrated by the extent to which we are still prepared to attribute to it all manner of feelings, mysteries and emotions, which do not have any basis in reality. Poets and songwriters have always talked about the lover's heart 'breaking' or 'aching' or even

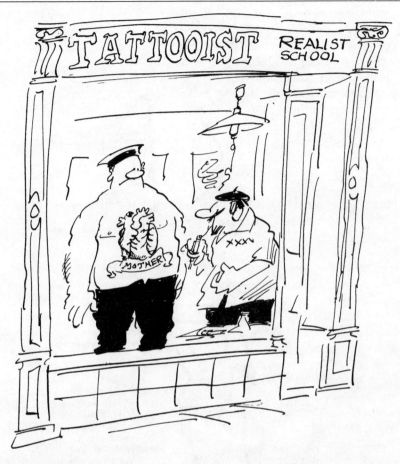

being left in San Francisco. It is still quite common to hear of someone dying of a 'broken heart'. Galen regarded the heart as a flame which heated the blood, an attitude which, although less romantic, still has a certain appeal. It was not until the great work of William Harvey in 1628 that the central role of the heart in propelling blood throughout the body was appreciated.

The Heart Itself

For our purposes we shall regard the heart simply as a pump – although admittedly an extraordinary one. It consists of a special type of muscle called the myocardium, and on average it beats or contracts 72 times per minute. As a rough approximation, it is about the size of a clenched fist and is situated in the centre of the chest extending to the left and with its

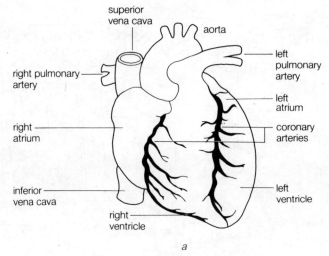

Figure 2.1 *a*

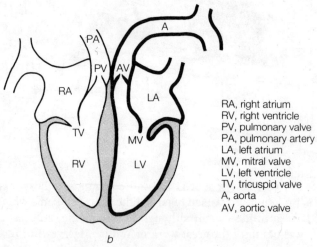

RA, right atrium
RV, right ventricle
PV, pulmonary valve
PA, pulmonary artery
LA, left atrium
MV, mitral valve
LV, left ventricle
TV, tricuspid valve
A, aorta
AV, aortic valve

Figure 2.1 *b*

apex extending almost to the left nipple. It is an extraordinary and beautifully constructed organ, which is also highly efficient. During the average lifetime it will beat an awesome $2\frac{1}{2}$–3 billion times.

The basic structure of the heart is shown in figure 2.1. The four chambers of the heart (two left, two right) are divided into the atria and the ventricles respectively. The function of the heart is to ensure the circulation of oxygen-enriched blood for use throughout the body. Oxygen is an essential requirement for the cells, without which the body would

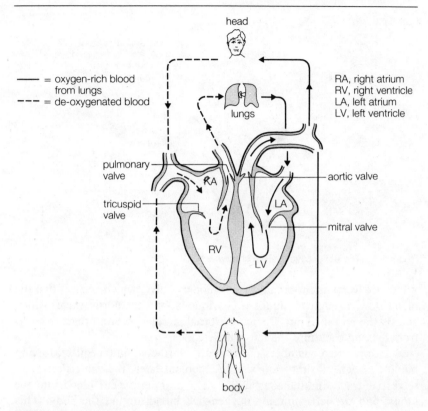

Figure 2.1 *c*

quickly die. When deprived of blood the brain, for example, will suffer irreversible damage within three or four minutes.

When the oxygen has been removed, the de-oxygenated blood returns to the heart via the veins. It enters the right atrium, and then passes into the right ventricle. From here it is pumped through the lungs, where via a complex series of reactions the blood is once again enriched with oxygen. This blood then drains into the left atrium and after passing through into the left ventricle is again pumped around the various parts of the body via the arteries. In general, therefore, arteries carry oxygen-rich blood away from the heart and the veins return oxygen-depleted blood to the heart.

There are a number of specialized valves in the heart which ensure that the blood passes in the right direction, and prevent any reflux of blood during cardiac contraction. The valve between the right atrium and ventricle is called the tricuspid (because it is composed of three leaflets of tissue), and the valve between the left atrium and ventricle is termed the mitral valve (because it is said to resemble a bishop's mitre). Two other

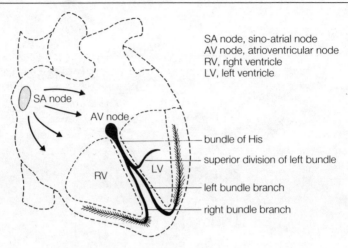

SA node, sino-atrial node
AV node, atrioventricular node
RV, right ventricle
LV, left ventricle

bundle of His
superior division of left bundle
left bundle branch
right bundle branch

Figure 2.2   The conductive system of the heart.

valves are worth mentioning; the pulmonary valve, which ensures that the blood flow through the lungs is continuous, and the aortic valve, which guards the entrance into the main arterial circulation and prevents blood from leaking back into the left ventricle.

The upper two chambers of the heart contract simultaneously, forcing blood through into the ventricles. A moment later, the ventricles themselves contract simultaneously, the right pumping spent blood into the lungs, and the left pumping oxygen-rich blood around the body. This sequence of events, the contraction of the atria and the subsequent contraction of the ventricles, is beautifully coordinated by a highly complex conducting system. In simple terms we can regard the conducting system for the pump as a series of electrical wires (figure 2.2). The impulse which initiates the heart beat is produced in the sino-atrial node, and is found high up in the right atrium. The sino-atrial node, or 'pacemaker', is made up of a highly specialized group of cells which send out a form of electrical impulse at regular intervals, usually about 72 per minute, which is the average resting heart rate. This impulse is conducted through the atria, causing them to contract. It is then received by the atrioventricular (AV) node and transmitted via the bundle of His. The latter has two main branches, the left and right bundle branches and the ventricle impulse is transmitted via these branches to the ventricles. After a slight delay, the ventricles themselves contract and there follows a pause, before the cycle is repeated again. The phase during which the chambers of the heart are actively contracting, first the atria, then a split second later the ventricles, is called systole. The phase during which the heart is resting between beats is termed diastole.

The Coronary Arteries

The heart, as with any other organ in the body, requires oxygen in order to function, and one might have expected, in view of its central role in blood distribution throughout the body, that the heart would have obtained its oxygen supply directly from the blood within its chambers. If that were the case, then the present epidemic of heart disease to which we are now referring would be eradicated. Unfortunately, this is not the case, and the blood supply to the heart is derived from two arteries, the right and left coronary arteries. In reality the left coronary artery divides into two shortly after its origin, so from a practical point of view there are three coronary vessels. They pass into the heart muscle and, after dividing into many smaller branches, supply blood and oxygen to the heart muscle (myocardium) (figure 2.3).

When we speak of 'coronary heart disease' it is disease in these three vessels to which we are referring. Coronary angiography, about which we shall have more to say later, is a specialized form of investigation in which a special dye is injected into the coronary arteries in order to make them visible under X-rays. A normal coronary angiogram is shown in plate 1. It shows clearly how the coronary arteries arise and how each branch then sub-divides into smaller branches.

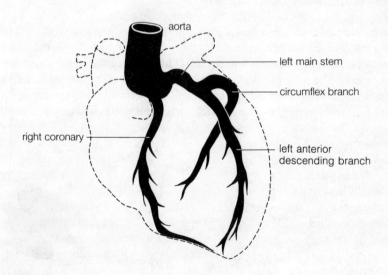

Figure 2.3   The arterial blood supply to the heart.

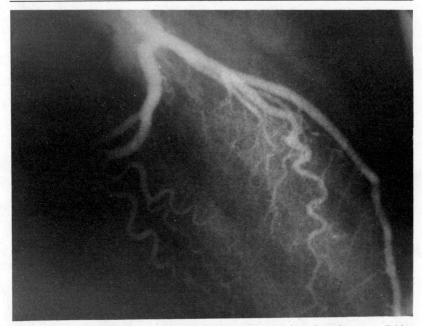

Plate 1   A normal coronary angiogram (left coronary artery). Note how the artery divides and sub-divides into tiny branches. The lining of the artery is smooth and clear.

What is Coronary Heart Disease?

In the normal state the arteries throughout the body are lined by a small layer of cells called the intima. In the newborn child the lining of the arteries is perfectly smooth and regular, allowing normal blood movement throughout the system. With advancing age, however, the lining of the arteries becomes thickened and irregular, a process which is primarily due to the deposition of certain fats, including cholesterol. This fatty 'plaque'

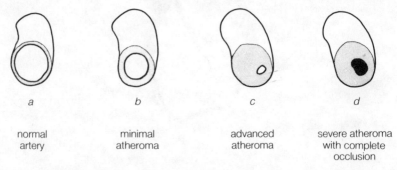

Figure 2.4   Arterial occlusion owing to atheroma.

is distributed throughout the blood vessel, although it is often very uneven in its distribution. Sometimes this plaque becomes very hard, or even calcified and brittle.

The chemistry involved in this deposition of fatty substances in the lining of the arteries is complex and need not concern us here. What is important is that the process will clearly interfere with normal blood flow, depending on the degree of hardening and narrowing, or occlusion, within the vessel (figure 2.4). This progressive furring up of the arteries is called 'arteriosclerosis' or 'atherosclerosis' and although it can and does occur in many vessels throughout the body, when it occurs in the coronary arteries themselves, the condition is referred to as coronary artery disease, coronary heart disease or ischaemic (i.e. lacking in blood) heart disease.

It will be evident to the reader that if the narrowing is slight, as in figure 2.4b, there will be no significant interference with the blood supplied to the heart and the patient will have no symptoms. Most people will have developed patches of atheroma in the arteries by the time they reach middle life and provided that the degree of narrowing produced does not materially interfere with the blood supply to the heart, it is of no consequence. This 'silting-up' process starts from a very early age and evidence of early atheromatous plaque can be found in the arteries of even very young children who have died from other causes. Progressive arterial narrowing and hardening is probably an inevitable accompaniment to old age. Most of us will have the disease to some extent, but unless it has progressed to the point where about 75 per cent of the normal diameter of the artery has been blocked, then we shall probably be free of symptoms and other ill effects.

In figure 2.4c it is clear that the process has extended even further and this situation has potentialy serious effects. When this narrowing begins to cause symptoms, we say that the patient has coronary heart disease. When the degree of narrowing has progressed to the point shown in figure 2.4c, there are three potential consequences – angina pectoris, heart attack or sudden death.

Angina Pectoris

In figure 2.4c the narrowing has progressed to the point where it significantly interferes with the blood supply to the heart. In this group of subjects, pain is likely to be a presenting complaint, although not inevitably. This is because when the heart rate increases in response to exercise the oxygen requirements of the heart increase and in normal circumstances there is increased blood flow through the arteries to supply the heart. When the artery is narrowed, the heart cannot derive sufficient blood, and therefore oxygen, to meet its demands. The result is pain, the correct term for which is angina pectoris ('pectoris' means 'of the chest') or simply angina. Very often the patient will not complain of symptoms at rest or even during moderate exertion. It is only when the exertion is of sufficient severity to provoke an increase in the oxygen requirements of the heart, which the narrowed vessel is unable to provide, that the pain ensues. In very severe disease, however, the pain may be provoked by even the smallest effort, for example walking or shaving.

The term 'angina' is derived from the Latin *angere*, which means to strangle, and a more apt description of the pain would not be found. Patients usually complain of a crushing, or 'gripping' sensation across the chest, or feeling as though a 'tight band' had been placed across the chest wall. This usually occurs on exertion, for example walking up a steep hill or hurrying for a bus. In most cases, when the patient stops the pain recedes within a few minutes. Sometimes there is an associated pain in the left arm or both arms, and often a sensation of 'pins and needles' in the fingers. Sometimes the pain may radiate into the throat or teeth and be accompanied by breathlessness and sweating of various degrees. This is the classic description of angina and elements of these symptoms can be found in most cases. However, there is a great deal of variation and patients may sometimes complain of only vague pains in the shoulder or hand, without any accompanying chest discomfort. Even in these atypical cases, however, when the activity precipitating the episode ceases, the demand for, and supply of oxygen to the heart returns to normal, and the pain recedes.

When the narrowing of the artery becomes very severe, e.g. to 90 or 95 per cent, the patient may complain of angina at rest, or when lying flat in bed at night (angina decubitus). This is a potentially lethal situation, since clearly at any time the blockage could become complete and a heart attack ensue. For this reason, this situation is termed (aptly), 'unstable' angina, in order to differentiate it from its more stable counterpart described above.

Finally there is another variant of angina which deserves a special mention. In some individuals, perhaps as many as 10 per cent, angina occurs in the presence of normal coronary arteries which show no evidence of the atheromatous plaque referred to previously. In these cases it is thought that temporary narrowing occurs due to a form of 'spasm' which may be provoked by a wide variety of stimuli, including exposure to low temperatures or even emotional stress. The mechanism is not clearly understood, but we now realize that coronary 'spasm' is an important phenomenon, and may cause symptoms or even cardiac damage in a significant number of individuals. Spasm can also occur in arteries which have evidence of atheromatous plaque, and it is clear that it is much more common than has hitherto been recognized.

Heart Attack (Myocardial Infarction)

The second major manifestation of coronary heart disease is acute myocardial infarction, or as it is more popularly termed, a heart attack. In figure 2.4*d* the diameter of lumen of the vessel has been completely blocked and this is usually due to a blood clot or thrombosis. When this process occurs in a coronary artery, we use the term 'coronary thrombosis' or heart attack; sometimes people refer simply to a 'coronary'. The correct medical term is 'myocardial infarction'.

What actually causes the thrombosis to occur at any given moment is not entirely clear, although we do have some idea as to the sequence of events which takes place. In figure 2.4*c* we can see that the blood vessel is about 90 per cent blocked and blood flow is clearly limited. The surface of the artery is irregular. Sometimes, because of a series of chemical reactions, the blood has a tendency to clot. If this occurs, the affected vessel will become completely blocked, as a result of which the area of heart muscle supplied by that vessel will suffer permanent damage. Clearly the larger the vessel involved, the greater the loss of heart muscle (myocardium) is likely to be. In figure 2.5, *a* indicates where a small artery has become blocked and consequently only a relatively small area of the heart has been damaged. In figure 2.5*b* the vessel is the left anterior descending artery, and the loss of myocardium in this situation is likely to be serious.

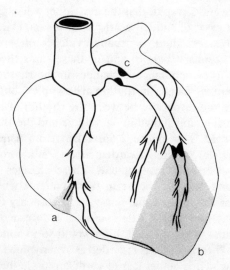

Figure 2.5   The heart attack (myocardial infarction). In (*a*) a relatively small artery has become blocked and a small area of the heart muscle has been lost. In (*b*) a larger vessel is involved and there is extensive loss of myocardium. A lesion at (*c*) implicates most of the heart and is potentially lethal.

In 2.5c the blockage is the left main stem itself and because the amount of myocardium at risk is so large, the situation is likely to be life-threatening.

This sequence of events, i.e. the furring up of the arteries, followed by a reduced blood flow and then thrombosis (clotting), which is thought to lead to a heart attack and loss of heart muscle, is a simplistic explanation for a highly complex process. Although this theory will serve our purpose, the reader should bear in mind that in some circumstances a heart attack (i.e. loss of myocardium), may occur without any evidence of thrombosis in the artery. For this reason some people have argued that the occurrence of a thrombosis in an artery is not a necessary pre-condition for producing a heart attack in a susceptible individual. Indeed, some have argued that a thrombosis in an artery is not the *cause* of a heart attack, but rather the consequence. The debate will certainly continue, but for the moment the idea of a blood clot causing the damage to the heart will suffice. In the next few years, further research into the role of coagulation (blood clotting) in causing heart attacks is likely to clarify the situation substantially.

Sudden Death

The last, and the most dramatic of the principal manifestations of coronary heart disease is that of sudden death. In this situation the blood supply through a major coronary artery is substantially reduced (for example, as in figure 2.5c) and, if a thrombosis occurs, the damage to the heart muscle may be so massive and so rapid, that the individual will expire within a few minutes. In most cases of sudden death, however, no evidence of thrombosis is found. Instead, there is usually evidence of severe generalized atheroma of the coronary arteries and in these cases the mechanism of death is thought to be spontaneous changes in the rhythm of the heart. These life-threatening changes in rhythm are complex, but the reader will readily appreciate the difference between the rhythm of the heart in the normal electrocardiograph shown in figure 2.6a and the abnormal rhythm illustrated in the ECG in figure 2.6b, taken from someone who had technically 'died' (i.e. suffered a cardiac arrest) on a coronary care unit, but who was successfully resuscitated. These changes in rhythm are usually sudden and may also occur in those patients who have actually suffered a heart attack in the usual sense, i.e. a coronary thrombosis.

The reader may now feel a little confused as to exactly what a heart attack is, and a final word of clarification would seem appropriate.

In most cases a 'heart attack' is regarded as synonymous with a 'myocardial infarction', which is actual loss of cardiac muscle due to a complete blockage in a coronary artery. Most cases of sudden death, however, are due to spontaneous disturbances in the normal rhythm of the heart, although the coronary arteries in most cases are diseased. Therefore, the

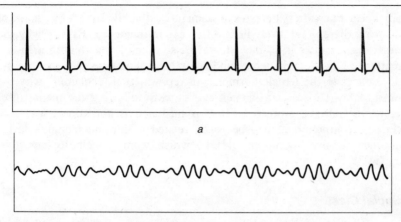

Figure 2.6   The electrocardiograph a, normal; b, abnormal rhythm leading to cardiac arrest.

term heart attack should include both those cases where cardiac damage is due to a thrombosis *and* those cases of suddent death due to spontaneous disturbances in rhythm due to underlying coronary artery disease.

Who Gets Coronary Heart Disease?

At the beginning of this chapter we emphasized that almost everyone is a potential victim of heart disease, irrespective of other factors such as age, sex and social class. There is a difference, however, in the incidence across these various sub-groups.

Age

Most deaths from heart disease occur in old age and the average age of death is approximately 74 years. It is important to observe that in England and Wales death from coronary heart disease also causes the annual loss of a million years of 'working life', with nearly 30,000 deaths in men under the age of 65. It is this 'premature' mortality which is so worrying and so devastating.

Sex

Coronary heart disease is the certified cause of death in 31 per cent of men and 23 per cent of women. Up to the age of 60 years the incidence of heart disease in women is substantially lower than in men, by a factor of five or six times. Thereafter, the rates in women rise quickly, so that by the age of 80 years there is relatively little difference in incidence. Exactly why the heart disease rates in women should be so much lower than in men is a matter of considerable debate and complexity. Some people attribute the differences to the female hormones of reproduction, explaining why the rates of heart disease in women rise quickly following the menopause. How this relative protective effect is mediated is not known with any certainty, although it may be partly related to the much higher levels of high density lipoprotein (HDL) which women seem to have (see appendix 1).

Social Class

In general heart disease kills large numbers of people from all social classes. There are, however, some differences in incidence between the various social groups which deserve special mention. Until the 1950s, heart disease tended to be more common among the higher social groups (i.e. groups 1 or 2). This picture has changed, and heart disease is now more common amongst the lower social groups, so that the mortality rates are about 30 per cent higher in the unskilled groups than for professional groups. Whether this is because the professional classes are, by virtue of better education, more susceptible to health education programmes with respect to diet and smoking is not confirmed.

Regional and National Variations

Apart from differences in age, sex and social class, there are also regional differences in mortality which are interesting. Death rates due to coronary heart disease are much higher in Scotland and Northern Ireland than in England and Wales, for both men and women.

International comparisons are instructive. The United Kingdom has not yet experienced the dramatic reductions in mortality from coronary heart disease which have occurred in a number of other 'Western' countries. The USA, Canada, Australia, New Zealand, Belgium and also Finland have shown substantial improvement during the past decade or so. Because of this, the United Kingdom's position in the international league table of heart disease is increasingly conspicuous. In 1978, the UK occupied three of the top five positions for men, and two of the top five positions for women (table 2.1). The tremendous reduction in heart disease mortality which has occurred during the past decade or so in the USA is of great significance. Between 1968 and 1978, sustained improvements were experienced in all age groups between 35 and 64 years and in 1978 the death rates fell below the corresponding rates in England and

Table 2.1   Coronary heart disease – the international 'top ten', 1978

Males		Females	
Country	Deaths per 100,000	Country	Deaths per 100,000
Finland	664	Scotland	256
Scotland	656	Northern Ireland	233
Northern Ireland	653	Israel	207
Eire	542	Eire	200
England & Wales	533	New Zealand	196
New Zealand	529	USA	187
USA	506	Australia	186
Australia	499	Finland	177
Canada	457	England & Wales	173
Denmark	443	Hungary	168

Figures show death rates per 100,000 for the age range 35–74 years.

Wales for the first time. The overall reduction in heart disease mortality was about 30 per cent and was estimated to have saved more than half a million lives (figure 2.7). Evidence would suggest that this improvement was due to improved health education regarding risk factors such as cigarette smoking and high blood pressure and the promotion of a more active lifestyle.

Latest figures (table 2.2) show that Scotland and England and Wales are still very high in the league table for coronary heart disease mortality,

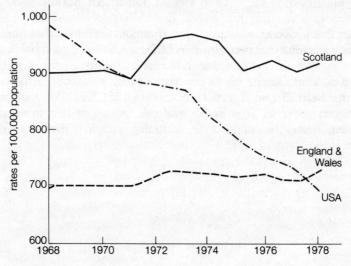

Figure 2.7   Deaths from coronary heart disease in males aged 55–64 years for the period 1968–78.

Table 2.2   Coronary heart disease – international comparison

Males			Females		
Year	Country	Deaths per 100,000	Year	Country	Deaths per 100,000
1981	N. Ireland	480	1981	N. Ireland	218
1984	Scotland	426	1984	Scotland	199
1983	Finland	414	1982	Sweden	173
1982	Sweden	377	1982	Denmark	172
1983	New Zealand	365	1983	New Zealand	170
1982	England & Wales	360	1982	United States	165
1982	Denmark	356	1983	Finland	164
1983	Australia	329	1983	Australia	162
1982	Canada	325	1982	Canada	162
1982	United States	324	1982	England & Wales	157
1984	West Germany	254	1983	Israel	147
1983	Israel	243	1984	West Germany	110
1981	France	112	1981	France	48
1984	Japan	61	1984	Japan	36

Figures show death rates per 100,000 of population for all age groups. The years indicated are those for which the most recent figures are available.

while the mortality rates for the USA, Finland and Australia are falling (note that table 2.1 shows death rates for the 35 to 74 age range, whereas table 2.2 shows death rates for all age groups).

That heart disease is essentially a disease of Western societies is graphically illustrated by the work of Dennis Burkitt. Dr Burkitt worked as a surgeon in a teaching hospital in East Africa for almost 20 years and during that period he accumulated an enormous amount of data from post-mortem examinations performed on Africans who had died at the hospital. His data showed that less than one case of coronary heart disease was found each year among the 98 per cent of patients who were African. The fact that heart disease is such a rare condition in Third World and under-developed countries is powerful evidence to suggest that much of our problem relates to our lifestyle, including smoking, diet and exercise patterns.

3

What Causes Heart Disease?

In the previous chapter we discussed the process by which the arteries become increasingly blocked with advancing age and saw how this can lead to symptoms of heart disease and even death. The key question, of course, is why should this process occur? In other words, what is the root cause of coronary heart disease?

Once again, the reader will not be surprised to learn that there is no simple answer. Indeed, it is not appropriate to talk of cause in the usually accepted sense of the word. Coronary heart disease is said to be a disease of 'multifactorial aetiology', that is, a disease in which a number of factors are known to be of importance in its causation, although none of these factors can be isolated as *the* cause. To illustrate the point, it is useful to consider a typical case history of a heart attack victim. By analysing the various factors involved, we can outline and discuss the most important points in the history.

Case history

CW was approaching his 48th birthday and had recently been promoted to the position of marketing director with a well-known electronics company. Although his promotion had resulted in a substantially improved salary and other benefits, CW found his new position a great deal more stressful than his previous job. He was involved in a lot of overseas travel, often away from home for long periods. His wife and two young children found this difficult to cope with, which also tended to make CW unhappy. He had not discussed the question of the new job with his wife in any detail – besides which, how could he have refused to take the position when it was offered to him? His predecessor had retired on health grounds, but CW was unaware of the exact circumstances by which the position had become available.

His medical history was unremarkable. He had suffered no serious childhood illnesses and had enjoyed good health for most of his life. At university he had been very active and played a great deal of rugby and soccer. For the past 20 years his activity patterns had decreased steadily, to the point where he had become completely sedentary. He smoked 40 cigarettes a day (his consumption had increased tremendously since taking on his new position), although he drank alcohol moderately. His weight had increased steadily during the last ten years and he was approximately 35 lb (16 kg) heavier than when he left university. Admittedly he did diet occasionally but the weight loss was short-lived and soon replaced. However, the family diet was a good one and his wife prided herself on providing a well-balanced diet, with plenty of meat, fresh vegetables and fruit.

CW's father had died at the age of 50 from a heart attack and he also had an elder brother, aged 51, with heart 'problems'. CW had never attended his own GP – he prided himself on never being ill, although he had intended for some time to go along for a 'check-up'.

One day in January, CW was preparing for a visit to Belgium, and rose at 7.00 am in order to travel to the airport. There had been heavy falls of snow for some days and on opening the bedroom curtains he quickly realized that his car would require some fairly extensive spadework to rescue it from the snow which had accumulated during the night.

After dressing quickly and grabbing a cup of coffee, CW set to work to dig out his car. He was already running late for his flight and would have to hurry. After two or three minutes of digging he was almost ready to drive away, when he noticed a vague ache in the centre of his chest. The pain was not particularly severe and after a few minutes had virtually disappeared altogether.

The traffic en-route to the airport was heavy and CW was becoming very anxious. In addition the pain in his chest had returned and was now, if anything, worse than previously. He managed to park his car in the airport car park and, carrying his suitcase, ran to the reception area. As he did so, the pain in his chest became very much more severe. He found himself feeling very breathless and was sweating profusely. The pain had spread into his left arm and was becoming much worse.

He found a chair and sat down for a few minutes even though his flight had already been called. At this point CW began to wonder whether he would be wiser to miss the flight and return home to rest. Still the contract which he was due to negotiate was so important that he felt duty bound to carry on with his journey, despite his feeling so unwell. Besides, it would not look very impressive if he lost this contract after only being in this new position for so short a time. People would begin to wonder whether they had made the correct decision to promote him in the first place. So, picking up his baggage and still wondering whether it was wise to continue, he headed for the check-in desk.

After a few yards, however, the pains in his chest became almost unbearable and just at the point where he was about to decide to seek some help the decision was made for him. He collapsed in the airport lounge and within a few minutes was heading at high speed towards one of the local hospitals. After being transferred from the ambulance to the casualty department he was transferred to the coronary care unit. A short while later electrocardiography confirmed that he had suffered a serious heart attack.

After a few weeks CW had recovered sufficiently to be allowed home. He is making excellent progress.

CW was one of the fortunate ones – he survived. His story is fairly typical and there are a number of factors we can identify in CW's history which are highly relevant to our discussion concerning the cause of heart disease.

First, he was clearly under a great deal of stress from a number of sources. We shall have much more to say about this later, but there is evidence that this form of stress may be important in contributing towards heart disease. Secondly, note his heavy cigarette consumption, and the fact that he had been physically sedentary for many years. Both these factors contribute to his development of coronary heart disease. It is clear that CW had become obese and he also had a strong family history of heart disease. CW had not seen his own family doctor for many years and so may well have been unaware of the hypertension (high blood pressure) which was subsequently found. Although he tried to eat a balanced diet, he was found on investigation to have a very high blood cholesterol level, and this was almost certainly a major contributing factor to his suffering a heart attack.

The factors we have isolated are known as the *conventional* coronary risk factors. Whilst we cannot identify one factor alone that will definitely lead to heart disease, we do know that the more factors that are present, the greater the likelihood of that individual's becoming a victim of heart disease.

The risk factors have been divided into two groups, major and minor. Before discussing these, it is worth pointing out that two major risk factors for heart disease are male sex and age, neither of which is amenable to change. The major risk factors are those that are known to have the strongest association with heart disease. They are as follows:

- Cigarette smoking
- High blood pressure (hypertension)
- High blood fats (hyperlipidaemia)
- Inactivity

Other risk factors, which are known to be of importance but where the evidence is less clear, are as follows:

- 'Stress'
- Obesity
- Diabetes
- Personality
- Hardness of tap water
- Family history
- Plasma fibrinogen

There is no consensus regarding which factor, or which combination of factors, is the most dangerous – 12 different cardiologists would probably give 12 different answers depending upon their experience. We shall consider each of the main risk factors in some detail, since although this book is primarily about the relationship between exercise and disease, the reader will be unable to understand the role of exercise in disease prevention without some understanding of how the disease is thought to occur in the first place.

The authors believe that the four most important factors in promoting the development of heart disease are:

- Cigarette smoking
- High blood fats (hyperlipidaemia)
- Hypertension (high blood pressure)
- Inactivity

These four factors are not necessarily listed in order of importance, although few physicians would dispute the contribution to premature death and disability made by cigarette smoking.

Cigarette Smoking

Smoking cigarettes is a slow form of suicide. At best it is playing Russian Roulette, only in this case there are three bullets in the chambers instead of one. Few people who are life-long smokers would survive unharmed. Death due to lung cancer, heart disease or chronic lung diseases such as bronchitis and emphysema are the future smokers can look forward to. Numerous studies have verified a clear relationship between cigarette smoking and heart disease. In general, male smokers have about twice the risk of non-smokers and there is a similar, although slightly smaller risk for women. However, the relative risk increases with the number of cigarettes smoked, so that for someone smoking 40 or more a day, the risk is increased fourfold. The risk is also a function of age, with younger patients being more susceptible to death than their older counterparts. Presumably this is due to the fact that those individuals who are especially susceptible to the adverse effects of smoking are eliminated from the population at an earlier stage in their lives, being survived by their more robust (or luckier) colleagues.

Exactly how cigarette smoking promotes the development of the 'furring-up' or atheroma in the coronary arteries is not clearly understood. There are about 4,000 chemical substances produced by a burning cigarette, and thus far attention has been directed only towards carbon monoxide and nicotine. There is some evidence that carbon monoxide in particular may play an important part in promoting the developing of the fatty plaque and encouraging the development of thrombosis. There is, in addition, a direct effect on the heart muscle itself.

Whatever the mechanism, there is little doubt that smoking is an important risk factor. Almost all readers should be aware that smoking cigarettes is harmful and we need hardly labour the point here. One or two points are worth making, however. First, if you do manage to stop smoking, the risk of death or disease begins to fall the moment you stop.

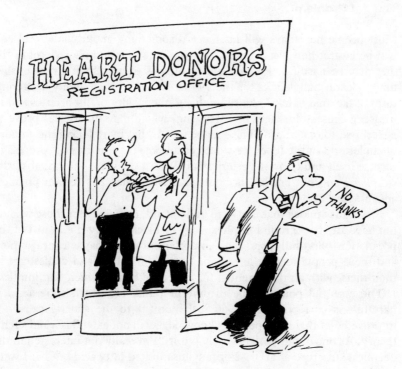

In other words, it is never too late to give up and the argument that 'I've been smoking for so long now that it isn't going to make any real difference' is simply another excuse to carry on with the habit.

Secondly, you should be aware that passive smoking (i.e. inhaling the smoke from someone else's cigarette) is also harmful. If your husband, wife or children are non-smokers, you will not be enhancing their health by continuing with the habit yourself.

If you are a woman, then it is worthwhile stating again that if you continue to smoke during pregnancy you run the risk of significantly damaging your unborn child. Damaging yourself is one thing, damaging someone else who has no choice in the matter is quite another. Pipe and cigar smoking are nothing like as harmful as cigarettes, although in certain groups of individuals they may increase the risk slightly. This may be due to differences in composition of the various kinds of tobacco smoke, the temperature at which the tobacco burns and the way in which the various kinds of tobaccos are cured. There is also probably a tendency to inhale pipe and cigar smoke less. Therefore, if you must smoke, they are certainly the better alternatives.

The Fat Problem

Most people nowadays will have heard something about cholesterol and will be aware, however vaguely, that too much fat and cholesterol in the diet may be harmful. Further questioning as to why such a relationship might exist usually elicits the theory that cholesterol is a highly dangerous form of fat, that 'sticks' like superglue to the insides of our arteries and in so doing causes blockages or narrowings which may themselves prove to be a threat to our health. The general idea is that by reducing the amount of cholesterol in the food, we would encourage the 'furring-up' process to reverse itself and clean the arteries out. Whilst the idea is almost absurdly simplistic and not entirely accurate, it nevertheless has certain practical advantages.

First, it is an idea that is easy to understand, especially for those who do not have any background in physiology or biochemistry (i.e., most of the population). Secondly, and most important of all, it may encourage more and more people to reduce the amount of animal fat and cholesterol in their diets, with all the potential for improved health which that implies.

The essential point in the theory, i.e., that too much cholesterol is harmful, is correct. It is of no real moment to the general cause for improved diet that most people's knowledge will not extend beyond such a theory. As one of our patients aptly put it, 'I'm really not interested in the chemical structure of HDL-2 or polyunsaturated fatty acids. What I want to know is, what should I spread on my toast in the mornings?' Later in the book we shall be giving you some practical and easy-to-follow advice with regard to diet, including what to spread on your toast. For the moment, we shall summarize the most important points with regard to what changes we as a society should be attempting to make in our eating habits.

There have, during the past decade or so, been numerous reports from many distinguished groups all over the world, including the World Health Organisation and the American Heart Association, making clear recommendations for change. In this country the National Advisory Committee on Nutrition Education (NACNE) report in 1983 and more recently the Committee on Medical Aspects of Food Policy (COMA) report, 1984, made very clear recommendations with regard to the British diet. These detailed reports are hardly bedtime reading, but it is possible to sum them up in one sentence that can be understood by everyone. It is, that we should *eat less animal fat, processed sugar and salt, and increase our intake of fibre*. That is the clearest statement possible from the mass of research data available. If you are quite happy to accept this as a general policy, all you need is to obtain some practical advice as to how you should go about implementing these simple changes. If you want to follow the argument further, we have included additional discussion of the fat problem in appendix 1.

Hypertension (High Blood Pressure)

High blood pressure, or hypertension to use the correct medical term, is a common and extremely important condition. At the present time it probably affects some 15–20 per cent of the adult population in Western countries, and since it is associated with premature death and disability, we clearly need to give it some detailed consideration.

The first thing to understand is that we all have a certain level of blood pressure; indeed it is essential to life. Many people seem confused about what is meant by 'blood pressure' and are under the impression that blood pressure at any level is harmful. Some are also confused about the meaning of 'hypertension', believing it to be due to some form of mental tension or stress. In this sense the term high blood pressure is possibly better, since it will avoid this confusion. However, your own doctor is likely to use the term 'hypertension', and you should have a clear understanding of what this means. In this discussion the terms 'hypertension' and 'high blood pressure' will be used interchangeably.

There are two components of blood pressure readings. When the heart is actively contracting and forcing blood through the arteries, the pressure within the system rises. Pressure measured during this period is called 'systolic' pressure. When the heart stops contracting, i.e. when it is resting between beats, the pressure falls to resting levels, and this pressure is termed 'diastolic' blood pressure. Blood pressure is usually expressed as one reading over the other, i.e. 120/80 (120 being the systolic and 80 being the diastolic pressure).

The accurate measurement of blood pressure has only been possible since the beginning of this century, with the advent of the sphygmoman-ometer. Most people will have seen this instrument at their doctor's surgery and will be familiar with the blood pressure cuff which is wrapped around the upper arm and inflated. The doctor then uses a stethoscope to listen over the artery as the cuff is deflated, and using this method he is able to identify the systolic and diastolic blood pressures. We express the pressure in millimetres of mercury, usually expressed as mmHg, since the instrument most commonly in use these days is the standard mercury sphygmomanometer. A normal blood pressure would therefore be expressed as 120/80 mmHg (Hg being the chemical symbol for mercury).

Having discussed briefly how blood pressure is measured and the units of measurement, we can now consider the question of what is a normal or an abnormal blood pressure. If we take a large number of individuals from the population and estimate their resting blood pressures, we shall find a considerable variation in our readings. The pressure will be distributed over a wide range, with some individuals having very high and others very low readings. Most of the samples will be somewhere between these two extremes (see figure 3.1).

It can be seen, therefore, that blood pressure readings form a wide spectrum and that in reality it is very difficult to pick one point on that

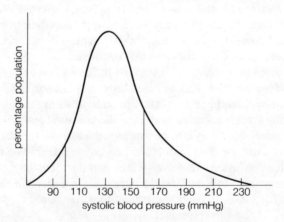

Figure 3.1   Blood pressure distribution in the 'normal' population. Most individuals have a systolic blood pressure between 100 and 160 mmHg, but a small percentage will have values above and below this range.

Table 3.1 Blood pressure classification

Normal	A blood pressure of 140/90 mmHg or lower
Borderline	A diastolic pressure between 90 and 95 mmHg
Mild hypertension	A diastolic pressure between 95 and 104 mmHg
Moderate hypertension	A diastolic pressure between 105 and 114 mmHg
Severe hypertension	A diastolic pressure of 115 mmHg or higher

spectrum, above which we would definitely regard a blood pressure as being abnormal. However, when we examine the statistics relating life expectancy to levels of blood pressure, it is clear that there is a linear relationship between long-term survival and levels of blood pressure, i.e. the higher your blood pressure, the less chance you have of living a normal lifespan. On the basis of this evidence, it is possible to define a level of blood pressure above which the probability of developing ill health is signficantly increased. We emphasize again, however, that this is not an *absolute* level above which we regard blood pressure as being abnormal. It is an arbitrary point at which the statistical evidence suggests a substantially increased risk from cardiovascular disease.

Since we need a point of reference, the World Health Organisation has defined normal blood pressure as a systolic pressure equal to or less than 140 mmHg, together with a diastolic value of 90 mmHg or less. If 140/90 is the upper limit of normal, what then do we regard as being abnormal or 'high' blood pressure? Again the figures are somewhat arbitrary, but those generally accepted as constituting hypertension are a sustained systolic pressure equal to or greater than 160 mmHg, and a diastolic level equal to or greater than 95 mmHg. Values falling between the normal figures and those which are regarded as abnormal are termed 'borderline'.

Elevated blood pressure is also classified as mild, moderate and severe. The position is summarized in table 3.1. Most practising physicians would accept these figures as reasonable working levels, although there is considerable controversy about the need to treat mild hypertension. Sir George Pickering, a distinguished worker in the area of hypertension, once defined high blood pressure as 'that blood pressure which is better treated than left alone'. Whilst correct, from a practical point of view this statement is not particularly helpful.

The reader should bear in mind one or two important points about blood pressure. First, we all have a certain level of blood pressure within our arterial system. If this were not the case, then the blood would be quite unable to move around the body in the normal manner. It is the *level* of that blood pressure which is important and which leads us to the concept of normal and abnormal blood pressure. It is also important to realize that there is a vast variation in blood pressure in normal individuals

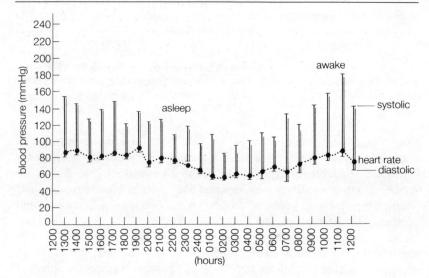

Figure 3.2   Variation in blood pressure and heart rate over a 24-hour period.

throughout a 24-hour period (see figure 3.2). Stress, eating, driving a car, exercise, etc., can all affect the blood pressure levels. This is why it is always important to make some attempt to standardize blood pressure readings by taking the pressure in the resting state, usually lying on a couch. Unless readings are standardized in some way, it is impossible to make meaningful comparisons.

Blood pressure during exercise may rise to quite high levels. The systolic pressure in particular may rise to 210 or 220 mmHg. Immediately following strenuous exertion, blood pressure values may fall quite substantially, usually below the 'resting' levels. It is clear, therefore, that the circumstances under which the blood pressure is estimated are extremely important.

So far as symptoms of high blood pressure are concerned, it is generally believed among the lay public that high blood pressure is associated with headaches, dizziness, lethargy and tiredness. In fact these symptoms are as common among those with normal blood pressure as those with hypertension, and cannot therefore be taken as a reliable indicator. Most people with high blood pressure have no symptoms at all and will therefore be totally unaware that this problem exists. This is why it is so important to have your doctor check your blood pressure fairly regularly.

We stated earlier that about 15–20 per cent of the adult population have high blood pressure. It must be understood, however, that this is an average figure and that hypertension is more common in older age groups. In the normal course of events blood pressure increases with age; therefore a value that we would regard as acceptable in a 70-year-old may be quite abnormal in a 30-year-old. In general, high blood pressure is very rare among children, becoming more common as the age advances. It is more common among young adult men than women of the same age range, but the incidence in both sexes is approximately the same in the 55–65 age range, with 35–40 per cent having higher than normal blood pressure levels.

What Causes High Blood Pressure?

In most cases of hypertension the cause cannot be identified and we refer to this form of high blood pressure as primary or 'essential' hypertension. In practice this accounts for the vast majority of patients with abnormally elevated blood pressure levels, perhaps as many as 90–95 per cent of cases. In the remaining 5 per cent or so there is an underlying cause which can be identified and these cases are referred to as 'secondary', i.e., the high blood pressure is secondary to some underlying cause. These patients need not concern us here but their high blood pressures may be related to kidney problems, rare disturbances of their hormone secreting system and, occasionally, to tumours. For practical purposes we can ignore this group, and concentrate on the group with essential hypertension, which is by far the most important.

Although we cannot identify any one cause, we do know that certain environmental factors can have a profound effect on our blood pressure readings. Some people have argued that salt is of great importance in promoting high levels of blood pressure in Western society, backing up their claims with evidence from countries where salt consumption is much lower than ours and where the incidence of high blood pressure is very substantially less than ours. There is also some experimental evidence that salt can cause high blood pressure in animals, although extrapolating these results to human beings clearly has limitations.

It is certainly a controversial issue, but there does now seem to be a consensus of opinion which recognizes that in a certain group of individuals high levels of salt in the diet may well promote unacceptably high blood pressure levels. It may well be that this 'salt-sensitive' group have a hereditary disposition to high blood pressure, in that they are unable to handle large amounts of sodium chloride. This may be due to a defect of the kidneys, although the exact mechanism is still a matter of continued research. Our view is that the salt intake of the population is unacceptably high and, in line with the recommendations of the previously mentioned NACNE report and, more recently, the COMA report, we would suggest that individuals should make every effort to reduce their salt consumption, perhaps by simply limiting their intake of added salt at the table. We believe this should apply to all individuals, irrespective of their blood pressure levels, since there is no evidence that moderate restrictions of this kind will do any harm and there is quite a lot of evidence to suggest that it may be of some benefit. Those subjects with established hypertension should certainly make every effort to reduce salt consumption, which, in combination with diet and weight loss, may well be sufficient to reduce blood pressure to normal levels.

Although we recognize that not all patients will respond equally, there is no question that some individuals respond to such dietary measures with quite dramatic improvements. It is unfortunate that there is at present no ready way of identifying such 'salt-sensitive' individuals other than by reducing salt intake in all hypertensives and monitoring the response. We shall have much more to say about the manipulation of blood pressure levels at a later stage.

Other factors known to be associated with high blood pressure are cigarette smoking and obesity, and again, much more will be said about these factors later. Smoking can substantially raise resting blood pressure levels, and obesity tends to be associated with raised blood pressure. In addition, such factors as 'stress', inactivity and fat intake may increase blood pressure levels. Alcohol consumption may also make a contribution to raised blood pressure levels, although this seems to apply mainly to heavy drinkers. Those who are more accustomed to more moderate levels of alcohol intake are probably not at risk.

It is clear, therefore, that raised blood pressure is associated with a number of environmental factors such as obesity, cigarette smoking, stress and alcohol. In addition, we should mention the contribution made by hereditary factors. In the case of hypertension this is difficult to assess because the fact that blood pressure varies so widely throughout the population, suggests that the genetic contribution to blood pressure levels is highly complex. It is certainly true that high blood pressure tends to run in families, but whether this is due to genetic factors or simply that children may tend to inherit the bad health habits of their parents, such as smoking and becoming obese, is difficult to establish. Even allowing for definite environmental risk factors which parents and children may have in common, however, there does seem to be some independent contribution to high blood pressure from genetic influences. In the case of twins for example, the blood pressures of identical twins are more alike than those of non-identical twins, and first-degree relatives of persons with high blood pressure have higher blood pressure than relatives of persons with normal blood pressure. In summary, therefore, if both your parents suffered with hypertension, then you will be more likely to develop similar problems yourself, although it does not necessarily mean that you will. In cases where the family history is very strong, it is obviously more important that you should have your own and your children's blood pressure checked regularly.

Although we have established that many factors, including genetic ones, have a part to play in the origin of hypertension, the exact mechanisms whereby these factors are mediated to produce increases in blood pressure are still not clear. The control of blood pressure within the body is highly complex, and the details need not concern us here. Suffice it to say that the kidney plays a central role in blood pressure control and that some disturbance of its normal regulatory ability contributes substantially to abnormally high levels of blood pressure.

Why Does Having High Blood Pressure Matter?

You may be wondering why such a long discussion of blood pressure is required and what implications increased levels of blood pressure have for the population in general. The short answer is that untreated high blood pressure is associated with a substantially reduced life expectancy, depending upon the levels in question. In the past there was a tendency to concentrate upon the levels of diastolic blood pressure in relation to premature disability and death, but it is now known that the systolic levels may also be a powerful predictor of subsequent heart disease. Among men with normal diastolic pressures but elevated systolic pressures there is a two-and-a-half fold increase in the death rate from heart disease when compared with individuals with normal systolic pressures. For nearly 70 years it has been known that patients with hypertension die prematurely.

The most common cause of death is heart disease and stroke, but kidney failure may also occur in some individuals. The largest population study of high blood pressure comes from the Framingham project in Massachusetts, USA, and these data confirm that people with high blood pressure are four times more likely to have heart failure, have three times as many heart attacks and seven times as many strokes as their normal counterparts. Small wonder therefore that insurance companies take great note of an individual's blood pressure when determining life insurance premiums.

With reference to coronary heart disease in particular, further data from the Framingham study suggest that the incidence of coronary disease rises by almost 20 per cent for each 10 mm increase in systolic pressure. At a systolic pressure of 160 mmHg the risk is about double that if the pressure were 110 mmHg. We also know that diastolic pressures exceeding 110 mmHg in middle age are associated with a one in five probability of death within five years if left untreated. Since we know that about 25 per cent of males in the age range 45–64 years may be classified as hypertensive, it is readily apparent that hypertension plays a major part in premature disability and death from cardiovascular disease.

Those individuals with elevated blood pressure are usually investigated to determine whether there is any 'target' organ damage before treatment begins. The kidneys, eyes and heart are referred to as the target organs, since they are the organs most at risk from the complications of high blood pressure. Kidney function is assessed biochemically and the urine is also tested for protein because damage to the kidneys results in abnormal protein loss. In addition, a chest X-ray and electrocardiography are performed to determine whether there is any evidence of enlargement of the heart, which can occur as a result of the elevation in blood pressure. Finally, it is also important to examine the eyes, since untreated high blood pressure may cause serious damage to the arteries in the eye and cause deterioration in vision.

When these investigations have been performed, consideration may then be given to management. Although we know that increased blood pressure levels are associated with increased mortality and heart attacks, strokes and kidney disease, the exact mechanism whereby high blood pressure causes damage to the arteries is not clearly established.

What Difference Does Treatment Make?

When the condition is identified and adequately treated the outlook is very much brighter. Evidence suggests that the incidence of complications described above is substantially reduced, and figure 3.3 illustrates this clearly. In other words, much of the premature death and disability associated with hypertensive disease is preventable. However, before it can be dealt with it must be identified, and in this country we need to become much more enthusiastic in attempting to identify the significant

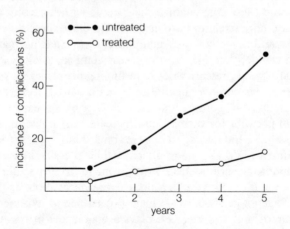

Figure 3.3   The effect of treatment on hypertension.

numbers of the population who have high blood pressure, but who are totally unaware of the fact. They are sitting on a time bomb, which may have catastrophic consequences.

In 1971, the Hypertension Study Group in the USA stated that '15–20 per cent of adults in the USA have hypertension . . . and the great majority are presently undetected, untreated or inadequately treated'. During the past decade, however, a concentrated and coordinated effort has been made to identify those at risk and the number of undiagnosed and untreated patients has been greatly reduced. This factor may be one of the most important in accounting for the tremendous reduction in deaths due to heart disease and strokes which the USA has experienced during that period. No such reduction has been seen in this country and there is a great need for a concentrated effort on a wide scale, to identify the hypertensives in our population. It is by no means uncommon to hear patients say they have never had their blood pressure estimated, or even in some cases that when they had requested a blood pressure measurement from their family doctor they were refused, or made to feel a nuisance. Such an attitude is inexcusable in the light of the available data.

Finally, we would emphasize again that there is no clear dividing line between normal and abnormal blood pressure. The relationship between blood pressure levels and long-term survival is quantitative. In other words, the lower your blood pressure the better your outlook and vice versa. The levels we have accepted as abnormal are those that are associated with an increased risk of developing a serious cardiovascular event.

One last point is that there is no such thing as a *low* blood pressure, occurring in a normal patient with no symptoms. In our own clinic patients often tell us someone has taken their blood pressure recently and been concerned because the pressure was low. These patients are often anxious about such a finding, thinking it may be every bit as significant as having high blood pressure. Provided a person has no symptoms, and does not have massive blood loss as a result of haemorrhage or burns or some other medical condition, the finding of a low pressure is of no significance, except that it is statistically associated with long-term survival!

Other Risk Factors

We have examined in some detail the relationship of heart disease to cigarette smoking, hyperlipidaemia (high blood fat levels) and hypertension because these three risk factors are generally agreed to be the most important. Many cardiologists would argue about which of the three is *the* most important, but few would doubt the overall importance of the 'big three'.

There are, however, a number of other risk factors of importance, but where the available evidence is perhaps not so conclusive. Hitherto, lack of exercise has generally been thought of as a minor factor, but there is now a substantial body of evidence to suggest that we may more appropriately regard it as belonging in the 'major' group, along with cigarette smoking, hyperlipidaemia and hypertension. We shall be presenting the evidence for this in chapter 4.

The other 'minor' risk factors, which we shall now discuss, are family history, obesity, personality, 'stress', diabetes, hardness of tap water and plasma fibrinogen.

Family History

There is no doubt that a strong family history of coronary heart disease is a significant risk factor and some workers would regard it as being of major importance. One of the problems in evaluating the role of genetics in heart disease is that environmental factors within families have a tendency to influence the incidence of disease. For example, if you are brought up in an environment where both parents smoke heavily and exist on a diet of chips, hamburgers and sausages, and where the only physical activity undertaken is changing the channel on the TV set, it is quite probable that you will grow to inherit the same health hazards. It is not always easy, therefore, to decide whether there is an inherited genetic tendency towards heart disease, or whether children simply inherit the bad habits of their parents. In addition, it may be that the genetic element is more closely related to the development of hypertension and hyperlipidaemia, which in turn, of course, is reflected in a higher incidence of coronary heart disease, there being a direct relationship between heart disease and heredity, i.e., the genetic element is mediated through other proved risk factors.

What one can say, however, is that if one or both of your parents died from coronary heart disease before the age of 55, then your chances of developing similar problems are increased. The better your genes to start with the less likely you are to develop problems. But the converse, although true, is by no means associated with the *inevitable* development of heart disease. In other words, even if your family history is strong, it does not mean to say that you will *necessarily* suffer premature disability or death yourself. There are a large number of other factors that would need to be taken into consideration, such as smoking habits, lifestyle, etc. If your family history is a bad one, it means you have one risk factor which you cannot alter, and which makes your attention to any other possible risk factors even more important.

Obesity

During the past 40 years there has been a progressive increase in the average weight of adults in Britain, and by 1981 more than 40 per cent of middle aged men and women were overweight. We shall have more to say about obesity later; for the present we must consider its relationship to heart disease. Unfortunately, it is difficult to disentangle the contribution of obesity to coronary heart disease from other risk factors with which it may be associated. For example, there is some evidence of a relationship between obesity and hyperlipidaemia, hypertension and diabetes, which in themselves are known to be significant risk factors for heart disease. Once again, therefore, it is not easy to determine the contribution that obesity by itself makes to disability or death.

We know there is an increased risk of coronary heart disease in the overweight, especially in younger men. In this younger group, mortality from heart disease was 30 per cent higher in those with a relative weight excess of 10 per cent. However, since as we have said obesity is associated with an increased risk of hyperlipidaemia, hypertension and diabetes mellitus, the excess risk for coronary heart disease may be mediated through these factors rather than by obesity *per se*. There is little evidence that obesity itself plays any major role in the development of heart disease.

Nevertheless, because of its associations (i.e., hypertension etc.), obesity is a definite risk factor which should be given serious consideration. Correction of excess weight often leads to substantial improvement in blood pressure and blood fats, and this in turn tends to reduce the risk. We shall see later that exercise has a major part to play in the treatment of obesity, and it should be borne in mind when prescribing exercise programmes for the grossly obese that arterial pressure often rises to extremely high levels in this group, who therefore need to be exercised with great care.

Personality

It has been recognized for many years that personality and behavioural traits may affect the outcome of disease in particular individuals. The possibility that personality may be associated specifically with coronary heart disease was first suggested in the 1930s and 1940s by Franz Alexander and Helen Flanders Dunbar, and subsequently by two Californian cardiologists, Mayer Friedman and Ray Rosenman. The latter described two forms of behavioural patterns in the subjects involved in their study, and these were designated Type 'A' and Type 'B' personalities.

The Type 'A' personality is characterized by intense ambition and competitive drive, constant preoccupation with deadlines, impatience with delay, time-consciousness, irritability and aggression. He is the sort of person who is forever looking at his watch and giving the impression that, although he is supposed to be having a conversation with you at present, he would actually rather be somewhere else, because he is already 45 minutes late. He may be tapping his pen on the desk top and saying 'Yes, yes' repeatedly, even though he may only have heard half the sentences being spoken to him. Bruhn and other workers describe the Type 'A' personality as exhibiting a Sisyphus pattern of behaviour – 'striving without sense of satisfaction or fulfilment', like the legendary Greek giant who was condemned by the gods to push a large stone up a hill, and who found that the stone always rolled back to the foot of the hill and he was forced to repeat the exercise over and over again.

The Type 'B' personality, as one might expect, is essentially the opposite. He is characterized by a low sense of ambition, little desire to compete, no real sense of time urgency and in general a far more phlegmatic or 'laid-back' attitude towards life.

There is evidence that Type 'A' personality may be much more susceptible to developing coronary heart disease than his more relaxed Type 'B' counterpart. A number of studies have tended to support this correlation, including two large epidemiological studies – the Western Collaborative Group Study and the Framingham Heart Study, both in the USA. Both studies showed a higher than expected incidence of coronary heart disease in those subjects exhibiting Type 'A' traits.

We believe that personality does have a part to play in the development of heart disease, but clearly the relationship cannot be claimed to be causal, i.e., Type 'A' personality may be associated with heart disease but does not inevitably cause it. Quantifying the risk in terms of other risk factors is difficult, although since Friedman and Rosenman claim that the incidence of heart disease is very much higher in Type 'A' than Type 'B' personalities, their own view is that it is of the same order of magnitude as a causative factor as hypertension and cigarette smoking.

The exact mechanism whereby personality influences the development of heart disease is not well understood, although one may postulate that it may act via the sympathetic nervous system, causing increased levels of catecholamines, adrenalin and noradrenalin, substances known to elevate blood pressure and blood lipids (fats). We have seen that increased blood pressure and lipid levels are major risk factors in the development of heart disease, and so once again it may be that personality traits are expressed through other well-defined risk factors to increase the risk in a particular individual. If this theory has any credibility, then one might expect to see high levels of adrenalin and noradrenalin in Type 'A' patients who are under stress. There is some evidence that this is the case, since although the levels of adrenalin and noradrenalin in the resting state were the same in both Type 'A' and Type 'B' subjects, when the same subjects were subjected to various forms of stress, there were much higher circulating levels of adrenalin and noradrenalin in Type 'A' subjects than in their Type 'B' counterparts. It is possible therefore that this mechanism may have a part to play in the association between personality type and coronary heart disease, although clearly the subject is enormously complex.

Since it is generally accepted that there is at least some contribution by personality traits to the development of heart disease, it might be asked whether there is any evidence that modifying behaviour would have a beneficial effect on the incidence of the disease. There is much research into this area at present, and we shall have to wait for the results of various trials. Preliminary findings, however, are encouraging and offer an interesting possibility for a more complete preventive approach in the future. Roskies and other workers in Quebec instituted a programme of Type 'A' behaviour modification in managers, and were able to demonstrate that such intervention strategies could bring about significant changes for the better in certain coronary risk factors.

We accept that personality has a contribution to make in terms of heart disease, although the extent of that risk and the extent of its contribution is not proved. Although we are currently researching into this area, clinical experience suggests that patients with established heart disease, or patients who can be shown to be in a high risk category in terms of conventional risk factors, do in fact have a wide range of personality traits and do not appear to conform to a clear identifiable sub-population.

Secondly, it will be readily apparent that it would be perfectly possible for a particular individual to display Type 'A' traits in one area of his life and Type 'B' traits in another. The accuracy of the Type 'A' trait assessment questionnaire, therefore, depends upon its ability to take into account these many factors. In appendix 2 we utilize a questionnaire, which is based upon the original used by Friedman and Rosenman, but which has been subsequently extended and validated by Professor Beech, at the Department of Clinical Psychology in Manchester. We believe it to be a useful guide to the assessment of Type 'A' traits and will allow the reader to gain some insight into his or her own personality rating.

Stress

The term 'stress' has now become almost as much in vogue as 'cholesterol' was in the late 1970s. Unfortunately, the term is not amenable to precise definition; it means different things to different people. There is an enormous amount of very confused thinking about stress and there is a general but mistaken notion that all forms of stress must, by definition, be harmful. This is by no means the case, and the subject is a good deal more complex than most people appreciate.

We all know what stress feels like and recognize that its origin may stem from a large number of sources in our environment. Most of us also appreciate that there is positive and negative stress and we are able to recognize the difference between the two. The stress of sitting in a traffic jam when we are already 20 minutes late for a crucially important business meeting, is very different from the stress a man might experience when waiting for his first child to be born. These qualitative differences in stress are very important, since they may not only be hazardous to health; they may also provide the impetus and determination to succeed in a particular venture or project.

We shall not be concerned here with the broader implications of stress, nor with underlying psychological mechanisms that have a part to play in our perception of potentially stressful situations. We are instead addressing the question of whether stressful life events can be shown to have any role in the development of heart disease. The short answer is that stress does appear to make a contribution and in some instances the onset of clinical symptoms can be clearly related to recent adverse life events, such as bereavement, divorce, unemployment, etc.

Prolonged stress may result in increases in blood pressure and blood fats, which, as we have seen, are strongly associated with heart disease. Obviously the question of personality is of great importance in understanding the effects of stress on any one individual, and there will be obvious differences in the way in which Type 'A' and Type 'B' personalities will react to any given level of stress. But what exactly is the relationship between personality type and stress? Although Type 'A' personalities are thought to have a higher incidence of heart disease, this may simply be due to the fact that in any given stressful situation they are more liable to react adversely than their Type 'B' counterparts. However, by far the most likely explanation is that the Type 'A' personality actively seeks out stressful situations and is therefore more subject to adverse life events. The Type 'A' personality is exceedingly ambitious and has a tendency to take on many projects at one time; an inevitable consequence of this is that the pressure and the complexity of his life increases. This is in sharp contrast to the Type 'B' personality whose relative lack of ambition and drive allows him to live his life in a quieter and much less complex way. It seems to us, therefore, that stress and personality are inextricably related, and one cannot adequately separate the personality type of an individual from his reaction to certain stressful circumstances.

All one can say is that stressful life events may certainly precipitate symptoms or even trigger a heart attack in some patients. There may even be important warning signs of chronic stress, such as increasing tiredness, irritability, inability to cope, symptoms which the person himself may not appreciate or which he dismisses as being of no significance. The failure to recognize such symptoms, which may be readily apparent to onlookers such as family or friends, may result in serious breakdown, both psychologically and physically. Dr Peter Nixon at the Charing Cross Hospital in London believes that many of us have lost the ability to recognize these warning signs, or else, because of social pressures, feel unable or unwilling to admit to them. Many people believe that to admit to one's inability to cope is an admission of weakness or defeat, and indicates a fundamental defect in our personality structure. Few people who found themselves promoted to a position within an organization would admit that they are in fact unable to cope with the new demands. Most of us would rather press on, under increasing pressure, than admit that the work is simply too much for us; indeed, we may strongly resent any such suggestion, even from close friends. Such chronic pressure and the unhappiness which springs from it, may have serious consequences for our long-term health and it is important that we try to recognize such symptoms in our own lives, and realize that there is a limit to the amount of stress with which we can safely cope.

Diabetes Mellitus

Studies on a variety of populations have shown a clear association between diabetes and coronary heart disease. In diabetics of all age ranges there is at least a twofold increase in the incidence of myocardial infarction (heart attack) compared with non-diabetics. This risk is markedly increased in younger diabetics and diabetic women are even more prone to coronary artery disease than diabetic men. The approximately twofold increase in the frequency of hyptertension among diabetics, especially adult females, may accentuate the risk and this relationship is probably associated with obesity.

Hardness of Water

There is some evidence that the hardness of tap water may be associated with coronary heart disease. There is a suggestion that undue softness of water may be associated with an increased risk of coronary heart disease, and an EEC directive to be implemented this year will require that the hardness of water should not be reduced artificially. The evidence for this association is not conclusive, although in the recent report of the Committee on Medical Aspects of Food Policy (COMA), it was suggested that individual members of the public who soften water in their own homes may wish to take the precaution of drinking unsoftened water.

Plasma Fibrinogen

Most coronary risk profiles include such factors as age, sex, blood pressure, lipid levels and cigarette smoking, and these have been discussed in some detail above. There is some evidence, however, that another substance in the blood, called fibrinogen, may also be an important predictor of future heart disease in some individuals. A number of controlled studies have suggested that this may be the case, and recent evidence from the Leigh Prospective Study by Stone and his colleagues supports the hypothesis.

Fibrinogen is a complex protein particle of the blood, which plays an important part in the process of blood coagulation, i.e., blood clotting. Since we know that the clotting of blood is an important mechanism in the development of coronary thrombosis or heart attack, it is clear that if there is an increased tendency of the blood to clot within an artery, an individual in whom such a tendency could be demonstrated might be expected to be at a greater risk of developing a heart attack.

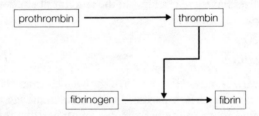

Figure 3.4   The Fibrinogen conversion process.

Figure 3.4 illustrates how fibrinogen is converted into fibrin under the influence of a substance called thrombin. Fibrin is the main framework of the blood clot within the body. Increased levels of fibrinogen may therefore indicate increased 'stickiness' of the blood, and therefore a greater tendency to clotting, causing a thrombosis.

Results thus far indicate that plasma fibrinogen is a significant, independent risk factor for coronary heart disease, which may be as important as raised blood pressure, high blood fats or cigarette smoking. Indeed, these other well-established risk factors may themselves influence the levels of fibrinogen in the blood, so once again the situation is probably more complex than first examination would suggest. It is probably true to say, however, that the addition of the plasma fibrinogen level to the standard coronary risk profile does significantly improve our ability to predict those apparently healthy individuals who are most at risk from developing a heart attack.

Inactivity

We have delayed the discussion of exercise in relation to heart disease until the next chapter because we believe there is evidence to suggest that patterns of activity can exert a profound effect on coronary risk profiles. For this reason, we consider that physical activity, or the lack of it, is a major factor in the development of coronary heart disease. It is at least as important as the factors we have already discussed in some detail.

The Overall Significance of Risk Factors

The reader will by now begin to realize that coronary heart disease and the factors responsible for its causation are enormously complex and difficult to unravel. The 11 factors we have examined have all been linked to heart disease in one way or another, although their relative importance is the subject of some controversy. In the document entitled 'Avoiding Heart Attacks' produced by the Department of Health and Social Security in 1981 the three factors given most prominence were cigarette smoking, high blood pressure and high blood fats. Few workers would argue that each of these factors exerts a powerful influence on the probability of developing coronary heart disease, irrespective of the presence or absence of other risk factors. Although we have accepted the importance of these three in our own discussion, we would also include a fourth, i.e., physical inactivity, which we believe to have a major influence on the development of heart disease. There is evidence that physical inactivity is an independent risk factor and that increasing patterns of activity may tend to influence favourably the manipulation of other known risk factors.

Some workers would regard a strong family history of heart disease as being of major importance, arguing that although the presence of conventional risk factors is of great importance, their occurrence does not account for all deaths from coronary heart disease. There are some individuals who have none of these conventional risks and yet become victims. Many of these people will be found to have a family history of heart disease, and presumably in this group, genetic influences are paramount. Equally there are many patients who display several risk factors, such as hypertension, hyperlipidaemia, obesity etc., who do not succumb. Presumably this apparent resistance derives from a low genetic susceptibility to the disease. There seems little doubt, therefore, that whilst the conventional risk factors are of major importance, genetic factors may to some extent determine the susceptibility of each individual. In other words, it is not a question of nature or nurture acting independently, but rather a combination of both, i.e., an interaction between a genetic tendency towards the disease and environmental factors such as cigarette-smoking and stress. We believe that lifestyle and habits are principal determinants of the development of coronary heart disease in any individual, although this tendency may be accentuated by an unquantifiable genetic factor.

It is also important to realize that risk factors in combination tend to compound the risk. For example, cigarette smoking in combination with high blood pressure more than doubles the risk, and the addition of raised blood cholesterol levels in combination with these two, increases the risk or coronary heart disease to more than eight times that for individuals without these risk factors. Some workers believe that the relative risk is grossly under-estimated. Khosla and his colleagues have calculated that in males aged 55–59 who smoke heavily and have abnormal levels of blood pressure and cholesterol, the risk of heart disease is 90 times that for men in the 40–44 yearage group who have none of these risk factors.

Whatever the truth, it is quite clear that the presence of multiple risk factors substantially increases the risk in any one individual. Since many of these risk factors can be shown to be independent of each other, attention must be paid to all potential factors, rather than concentrating on one to the exclusion of the others. This is an important point and one to which we shall be returning later in our discussion.

The Investigation of Heart Disease

Whilst we hope that readers of this book will be able to avoid problems related to heart disease, we recognize that many individuals will already have become its victims. In concluding this chapter, we shall describe briefly the more common techniques of investigating heart disease. Most individuals who have symptoms of heart disease, e.g. chest pain on exertion or breathlessness, will undergo a certain group of standard tests to help establish a diagnosis. These tests are as follows.

Chest X-ray

This enables the detection of certain abnormalities of the heart and lungs, which may give clues as to the correct diagnosis. Features visible on X-ray, such as enlargement of the heart in general, or selective enlargement of particular chambers within the heart, provide valuable information which may suggest the direction that further investigations should take. In many patients with coronary heart disease, however, the chest X-ray may be perfectly normal.

Electrocardiography (ECG)

It takes many years of practice to become proficient at reading an electro-cardiograph. In essence, an ECG is simply an expression of the electrical activity in the heart when looked at from several directions. Most ECGs nowadays are standard 12-lead recordings, that is, they are made by recording through 10 electrodes placed on the patient's trunk. An example of a normal ECG trace is shown in figure 3.5.

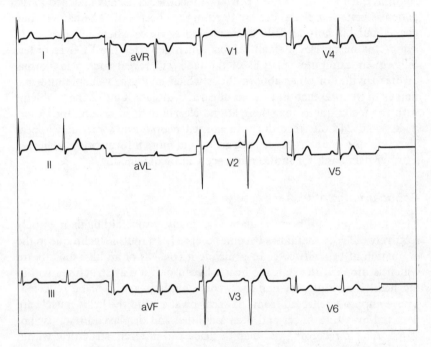

Figure 3.5   A standard 12–lead electrocardiograph.

When an individual suffers damage to the heart as a result of coronary disease, certain changes may be revealed in the ECG which indicate the extent and site of the damage. It is not important for the reader to understand the mechanisms of such electrical changes, but only to appreciate that a difference in the ECG pattern is readily apparent on inspection. The ECG may also give information about the rhythm of the heart and this may be of great importance in evaluating patients with coronary disease.

In patients with severe heart disease who have suffered one or more heart attacks, and who have therefore damaged their heart muscle irreversibly, the ECG is usually, but by no means always, abnormal. In cases where an individual has symptoms of heart disease, for example angina, but who has not actually suffered definite myocardial damage, the ECG may well be entirely normal.

24-Hour Ambulatory Electrocardiography

This technique is useful in evaluating cardiac function, especially the heart rhythm, during a full 24-hour period. A recorder is usually attached to the patient's belt, and electrodes are fixed to the chest wall. The patient then goes about his normal daily business and at times when he experiences symptoms he presses a small button which activates the ECG recorder. Subsequent computer analysis of the tape will reveal runs of abnormal cardiac rhythm or other abnormalities which may give valuable information as to the presence and extent of cardiac disease. One of the problems with the technique is that there are no clearly defined criteria for abnormality and 24-hour recordings in normal people can sometimes appear alarming. No doubt as experience grows and more information is collected a firmer data bank for future reference will be obtained.

Echocardiography

This technique has been available for many years, although it is only relatively recently that it has become accepted as a routine technique in the evaluation of heart disease. In principle it consists of an ultrasonic beam which is directed through the heart. Because different structures within the heart have different densities, some of the waves will be reflected. These impulses reflected from the cardiac valves and the heart muscle are detected by a transducer and then amplified and displayed on an oscilloscope. A strip recording can then be made and different structures within the heart can be clearly identified.

Echocardiography is a non-invasive (i.e. does not involve the introduction of needles or catheters into the body) and therefore painless technique. In experienced hands it takes only a few minutes to perform and gives valuable information concerning the function of the heart valves and also the condition of the heart muscle. It is, however, extremely expensive, and not yet part of the routine investigative equipment available to most hospitals.

Exercise Electrocardiography

This technique, otherwise known as exercise stress testing, or functional/ diagnostic exercise testing, is a powerful tool that is now playing a major role in the detection and evaluation of coronary heart disease. The corner-stone of modern stress testing is the empirical discovery that exercise in patients with coronary disease produces changes in the electrocardio-graph. This observation was made more than 50 years ago and during this period the technique and the theory behind it have been substantially refined. The advent of microprocessors has facilitated the development of computerized testing systems with a high degree of accuracy and precision.

The patient is first prepared for the exercise test by having the skin of the chest wall cleaned vigorously with alcohol or surgical spirit, having first shaved the area if this is thought necessary. The electrodes are then applied to the chest wall according to strictly defined criteria and a resting electrocardiograph is taken (see plate 2). The patient is then placed on a treadmill or a bicycle ergometer (stationary exercise bicycle) and the exercise is commenced. There are many different exercise protocols avail-able and specific protocols are used depending upon the situation. In our own laboratory we use a modification of the Balke protocol (named after Bruno Balke, who first designed the procedure). The subject is walked at a constant speed for six minutes with the slope of the treadmill increasing at two minute intervals.

Blood pressure measurement is carried out at regular intervals through-out the test and, in our laboratory we are also able to measure various exercise respiratory variables, such as maximum oxygen consumption and

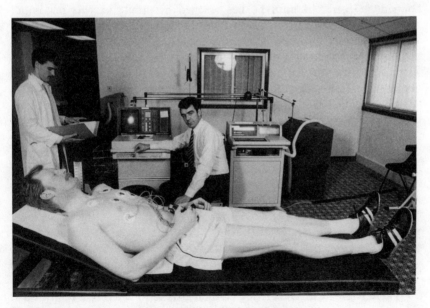

Plate 2   A subject prepared for an exercise electrocardiograph.

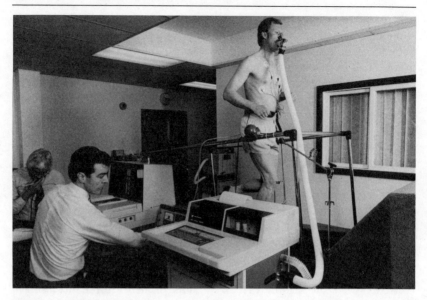

Plate 3   A subject undergoing a functional/diagnostic exercise stress test.

ventilation etc. (see chapter 5). At each stage during the test the electrocardiograph is scrutinized by a physician with cardiological experience and unless there are any specific contraindications to the test continuing, the patient is exercised until he has reached his limit, i.e. his maximum capacity. The test is thus limited by the patient's capacity to continue rather than by any pre-set criteria, i.e. it is symptom-limited (plate 3).

Following the test the subject will lie down for a further period of six to eight minutes, during which we continue to monitor the ECG. The recovery period is extremely important, since certain changes suggestive of underlying heart disease may not appear during the exercise phase itself, but during the recovery period.

The criteria for regarding an exercise test as being positive, i.e. predicting underlying heart disease, are varied and complex. The important changes to note are those that occur in what is known as the ST segment of the ECG recording. In figure 3.6 a normal exercise ECG pattern is illustrated, showing that the trace in the ST segment is level throughout. In the second ECG in figure 3.6 it is clear that the trace in the ST segment has become considerably depressed below the baseline, in this case to about 4 mm. This recording was taken from a subject who had no symptoms of any kind but who on further investigation was shown to have inoperable coronary artery disease.

There is great dispute among cardiologists as to whether a positive test should be regarded as one in which the ST segment is depressed 1, 1.5 or 2 mm below the baseline, and clearly these criteria will determine the

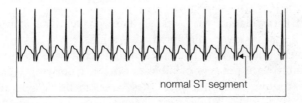

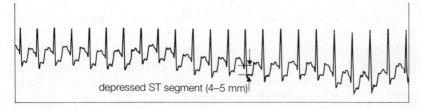

Figure 3.6 The exercise electrocardiograph.

incidence of false-positive and false-negative tests. In the simple terms this means that there is a danger that some people will be told they have coronary heart disease when they do not and some will be told that they have no evidence of underlying heart disease when in fact they have. It is this apparent failure of the exercise test to be 100 per cent reliable that has led to so much controversy in medical circles. There is little argument that when the test is applied to a population under the age of 35 years who have none of the conventional coronary risk factors that the test has a limited predictive value (this means that there may be a significant number of false-positives), and it is this worry that has led many physicians to criticize the usefulness of the exercise ECG in predicting coronary heart disease. This is unfortunate and in our view has led to the application of the test being far more restricted than workers in the field would have hoped. It stems from a failure of many doctors to understand the application of exercise testing, and the theory upon which it is based.

The fact is that in our population at present, the incidence of underlying coronary heart disease is high. We have seen that the vast majority of individuals in this society have at least some degree of atheroma in their coronary arteries, and that the extent of this process determines the risk of dying, or being prematurely disabled by a heart attack. We also know that the likelihood of significnt narrowing of the arteries being present is substantially increased when the conventional coronary risk factors are present. We also know that the more risk factors an individual has, the more likely he is to have a life-threatening narrowing of his coronary arteries. We believe that when the technique of exercise testing is properly applied to a population with one or more conventional coronary risk factors, the test has a very high predictive value.

In our own series we have documented significant ECG abnormalities in approximately eight per cent of subjects who have no symptoms and who attend for routine screening and fitness assessment. When the data is analysed it is clear that 80 per cent of the group with positive tests have one or more conventional risk factors, and many of them have two or more.

We shall have more to say about the value of exercise testing in chapter 10 but there is no question that it has a central role to play in the investigation of heart disease. Moreover, because it is a relatively safe procedure (1 death for every 10,000 hours of testing), it could be applied on a wide basis. We appreciate that the costs of such a programme would be enormous and it would also be impracticable. Nevertheless, there is, in our opinion, a sub-group of patients who can be regarded as at high risk, and who would benefit from an exercise stress test prior to becoming involved in exercise programmes.

Coronary Angiography

In most cases where the exercise test is unequivocally positive the next investigation is a coronary angiogram. This is an 'invasive' procedure; it involves placing a large needle into an artery (usully in the groin) and, after threading a catheter through the needle into the heart, a special dye is injected, X-ray pictures are taken and these illustrate accurately the condition of the coronary arteries. This is of great advantage in estimating the extent of the disease in any patient, and it is always performed before heart surgery. Because it allows visualization of the arteries themselves, surgical procedures can be planned with a high degree of accuracy.

Prevention Not Cure

Most of the investigations described above are routinely available in large hospitals, although there are other more sophisitcated means of investigation being developed now, which will undoubtedly have a greater part to play in the near future. Much more accurate information regarding the state of the coronary arteries and the function of the heart itself will become possible and the selection of those patients who would benefit most from surgery will be rationalized.

This is not a book about the treatment of heart disease or indeed about the diagnosis of this condition. It is about the ways in which lack of exercise and related risk factors can act in concert to disable or kill many thousands of people prematurely. Many people will already have evidence of this disease and we believe that much can be done to optimize their psychological and physical condition. Drugs and coronary 'bypass' surgery have enormously improved the lot of those people with established disease.

However, we must not let ourselves be seduced into believing that technology, however sophisticated, can solve the problem. The most effective way to deal with this disease is to *prevent* it. The coronary arteries of thousands of people are becoming blocked and causing problems. Unblocking them is extremely difficult and hazardous, and for most people impossible. How much better and more effective to prevent the process in the first place. Blocked coronary arteries have given the cardiologists a seemingly unremitting workload. Instead of adding to it, we should be directing our efforts towards means of prevention, both for ourselves and for our children.

4

The Exercise Factor

In previous chapters we have examined the role of various risk factors in the development of so-called 'Western diseases', particularly coronary heart disease. Lack of physical activity has been identified as but one factor among the many that have been implicated, and the 'multifactorial' nature of coronary heart disease has been emphasized. Cigarette smoking, high blood pressure and high blood fats (cholesterol) are generally accepted as major conventional risk factors for heart disease and, although it is accepted that lack of physical activity is a significant factor, it has not in general been accepted as being of major importance.

In this section we shall examine the role of exercise in disease prevention in more detail and argue that lack of physical exercise should be regarded as a major factor in the development of heart disease. Indeed, we believe there is good reason to regard regular physical activity as the cornerstone of good health policy.

Our argument is based upon the evidence from two main lines of inquiry. First, the epidemiological evidence which has been accumulating for the past 30 years or so suggests that exercise has a major part to play in disease prevention. Secondly, the evidence concerning the physiological and biochemical changes that occur as a result of regular exercise and, in particular, the way in which they may modify the known risk factors for heart disease, provides a basis for understanding *how* exercise exerts its beneficial effects. Because exercise is able to modify many of the conventional coronary risk factors, we shall argue that it should occupy a central position in primary disease prevention.

Since the time of the Ancient Greeks, physical exercise has tended to be associated with good health. Man has pursued recreational and competitive sport, satisfied that a fit individual was synonymous with a healthy individual. There was no scientific evidence to substantiate this relationship and indeed we shall see later that this is not necessarily true. It is certainly possible to be in sound health but unfit and equally possible to be very fit but unhealthy.

In the early part of this century, exercise came under attack in the form of the 'rate-of-living theory'. According to this theory, the greater the rate of energy expenditure and oxygen utilization, the shorter the lifespan. In other words, the more active you are, the shorter your potential lifespan. This is an extremely mechanistic view, but it cast some doubts on the value of physical exercise, and as recently as 1970 some scientists were of the opinion that exercise represented a stress to the body, with long-term harmful effects similar to those of infections, trauma and other disease processes. These theories have gradually lost their influence on society as the reduction in physical activity during work and leisure has become associated with the increase in coronary heart disease that now makes it the biggest single killer in society.

Man still retains an admirable capacity for exercise. He is able to attain speeds of 28 mph, jump more than 29 ft, climb the highest mountains and run a marathon in 2 hours 8 minutes. But these great gifts are given to few, and the individuals capable of these feats are idolized by thousands of sedentary spectators. We have become a nation of watchers, content to observe the gladiators of sport expend more energy in 90 minutes than most of us use in a day. A small proportion of the population is very highly active, but the remainder are almost completely sedentary. In health terms it would be far better if we were to spread the total energy expenditure during exercise evenly across the whole population, so that virtually everyone could be classified as *moderately* active, rather than having a small group involved in extremely high levels of exercise with the remainder of the population doing virtually nothing.

Most adults today believe that their physical condition is essentially unchangeable, and they long ago gave up the idea of achieving fitness and strength again, if indeed they ever possessed these qualities. A significant component of this appears to be the fear of ridicule and embarrassment at what would amount to a public admission of their poor physical condition. Many of those who attend our laboratory opt to take exercise late at night (despite advice to the contrary) for fear of being seen by their neighbours. Most people, however, resign themselves to remaining inactive, and decide to stay overweight, weak and clumsy. It is the soft option: few people realize how easy it is to achieve a reasonable standard of fitness, and how little time it takes.

We are persuaded that the weight of scientific evidence now available supports a general recommendation that the whole population should become much more physically active than it is at present. This does not mean that we should all aim to become marathon runners, become obsessional about exercise, or ignore other equally important aspects of our lifestyles. It simply means that we should try to reclassify ourselves as moderately active as opposed to totally sedentary.

Before examining some of the evidence, we wish to make it clear that if you are awaiting absolute proof of the beneficial properties of exercise, you will almost certainly be doomed to a life of inactivity, because absolute proof will not be available for the next 50 years. The reason for this will become clear as we explore the present scientific data and come to understand some of the very considerable difficulties encountered in making epidemiological studies of this kind. Despite this, we believe that the weight of evidence available at present strongly supports the hypothesis that regular exercise has a powerful preventive role in coronary heart disease. The lack of absolute proof should not preclude our taking concerted action to implement exercise programmes on a wide scale. Neither does it suggest that absolute proof will never be available. It simply means that absolutely conclusive scientific evidence is not available at present, mainly due to the difficulties and complexities encountered in this area of study.

We should not find this disturbing. All science is probability, and this applies nowhere more clearly than in medicine. We are not dealing with chemical experiments or equations which follow pre-determined laws. We are dealing with people, and in epidemiology we are dealing with populations of people. The number of possible variations within a population is infinite, and this is why the construction of the perfect epidemiological study is never achieved (and never will be). We have to be content with broader indications of trends and patterns. There will always be exceptions: they should not, however, distract our attention from the main body of evidence.

Epidemiology – a Review of the Data

Epidemiology is the study of disease patterns and trends within populations, and since the early 1950s epidemiological studies related to heart disease have been conducted in many countries. In general, these investigations have examined activity patterns within a community and compared the frequency of coronary heart disease in the most active with those in the moderately active and sedentary. In the early 1950s and 1960s the energy requirements within and between industrial occupations were substantial, and this provided a sound base for long-term studies of five to 20 years. As technology has progressed, the physical requirements in many occupations have been substantially reduced or removed altogether, and people have become much more reliant upon exercise in leisure time as a means of maintaining fitness. In keeping with this trend, we shall see that many of the studies have focused upon the relationship between heart disease and leisure-time activity, rather than being concerned with occupational activity.

We shall now review some of the studies conducted during the past 30 years, which show a relationship between activity patterns and the incidence of coronary heart disease. Our examination of the evidence is hardly comprehensive, since the literature is extensive. However, we believe that we are presenting a fair cross-section of the data available, including those studies which do not indicate any significnt relationship between heart disease and exercise.

We shall go on to discuss some of the criticisms of the studies we have considered, and formulate what we believe to be a reasonable conclusion.

Morris and Co-workers (1953) – the London Transport Study

The first large-scale study relating physical activity to coronary heart disease is the now famous and often quoted study of London Transport workers by Morris and others which was published in 1953. The occurrence of heart disease in the drivers and conductors of the Central 'red' buses, the drivers and conductors of trams and trolleybuses, and the motormen and guards on the underground railways was observed. In all, about 31,000 men aged 35–64 were studied, two years' data being obtained for the workers on the Central buses, trams and trolleybuses, and one year's data on the guards and motormen.

The essential difference between these groups in terms of physical activity patterns is obvious. The conductors are far more active than the drivers, and the climbing up and down the stairs of the buses, together with the walking up and down the length of the vehicle, amounted to a very considerable energy expenditure. By comparison, the drivers' job was essentially sedentary.

Analysis of the data showed that the conductors had 50 per cent fewer heart attacks when compared with the drivers. In addition, drivers suffered twice as many fatal heart attacks as conductors. Not only did the conductors have less coronary disease than the drivers, but what disease they did have appeared later in life and was less severe.

The data on the underground railwaymen showed a pattern of disease similar to the road vehicle drivers. This group of workers' job closely resembles the essentially sedentary occupation of the bus drivers, and so, if exercise is an important factor in disease prevention, it is hardly surprising that this essentially sedentary group should have the same incidence of heart disease as the bus drivers.

This study was criticized on a number of counts. First, it was argued, the men who were drivers may have 'self-selected' themselves for that particular occupation. In other words, something in their early experience and their constitution led them to choose that occupation, and along with this may have gone a hereditary predisposition to develop heart disease. This charge of self-selection is one which occurs time and time again in criticizing epidemiological studies. In the case of Morris' study, it could not be refuted, but neither could it be proved. There is absolutely no evidence to support the view that some factor present in the make-up of bus drivers led them to choose to be bus drivers, and that along with this there also happened to be a predisposition towards heart disease. It is quite possible to pose the alternative question, which is why should bus drivers be any different constitutionally or genetically from the rest of us?

The study was further attacked because it did not take into account other coronary risk factors such as obesity, stress, blood pressure and blood cholesterol. It was argued that the reason why the drivers displayed a much higher incidence of coronary disease than the conductors was simply that they tended to be fatter, and hence have higher blood pressures and blood fats than their colleagues. Thus, the apparent discrepancy in heart attack rates may have had nothing at all to do with the activity patterns of the conductors and drivers. As a matter of fact, a retrospective analysis conducted by Morris and his colleagues entitled, 'Physique of London busmen: the epidemiology of uniforms', confirmed that bus drivers tended to be more obese than the conductors when joining the service. This was found by analysing the waistband size of the uniforms provided for them, and it was found that the drivers were fitted with trousers that were at least 1 inch greater in waist circumference than the conductors. The drivers were also found to have higher serum cholesterol and blood pressure levels. Since the drivers were clearly not in the same physical condition as the conductors when they joined, it was difficult to determine whether exercise played a significant role in reducing the number of heart attacks, or whether the reduction was the result of these initial differences. This was an obvious fault in the study, and it precluded any firm conclusions being reached concerning the possible protective effect of exercise.

There is, however, another view which seems perfectly plausible, and which tends to support Morris' original hypothesis. It may be that the differences in the physical condition of the drivers and conductors at the time of joining the transport service were due to activity patterns carried out some time before taking up their new occupations. In other words, conductors may have been relatively thinner and with lower blood fats and blood pressures because they already had high activity patterns. The converse may be true of the drivers, for whom sitting in a cab all day may simply have been an extension of an already sedentary lifestyle. If this were true, then the exercise/heart disease hypothesis would be supported. Unfortunately, there are no data concerning the activity patterns of the men before they joined, so such an explanation is purely speculative.

Despite the criticisms, however, the study was nevertheless a vitally important landmark in the field. Morris and his colleagues had tested an important hypothesis and found evidence to support it. The fact that the evidence could not be regarded as conclusive is hardly relevant now. It was this pioneering work which opened the floodgates during the next 30 years for large-scale epidemiological studies examining the relationship between activity patterns and heart disease, and Morris himself was to contribute in no small measure to much of the research that was to follow.

Morris and Co-workers (1953) – the Postal Workers and Civic Servants Study

In the same paper in which Morris had reported the investigation of heart disease in the London Transport workers, he also reported a study of heart disease in postal workers and civil servants. This work had been carried out in parallel with the transport workers' study.

Male postal workers, together with clerical and executive grades in the civil service, were studied: a total of 110,000 men, most of whom were studied for two years. Physical exertion at work for the postmen was greater than that for the other grades studied, and the data obtained showed that the total incidence of heart disease in postmen is lower than

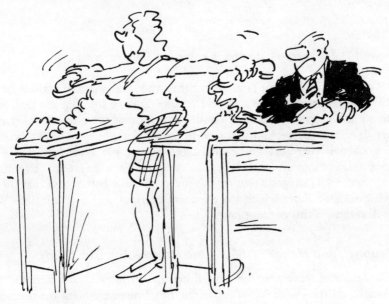

that in the sedentary grades. In addition, what coronary disease the postmen do have is less severe than that found in those with clerical and other sedentary occupations. Thus, the findings in this parallel study were broadly in agreement with those of the transport workers' study. Once again, therefore, the basic hypothesis that exercise exerted a protective effect against heart disease in middle-aged men was supported.

Zukel and Co-workers (1959) – The Dakota Farmers Study

In 1959, Zukel and colleagues published the results from a one-year study in North Dakota, comparing the incidence of heart disease among farmers and non-farmers living in the same area. The sample was graded according to the number of hours of physical activity performed each day. The results showed quite clearly that farmers had lower rates of heart disease than non-farmers, and the difference was attributed to smoking and physical activity.

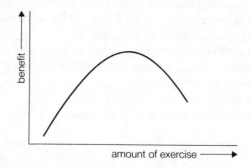

Figure 4.1   The inverted U hypothesis – more exercise is not better.

One other interesting point about this study was that the highest rates for coronary heart disease were seen among those performing less than one hour's activity per day, and also in those performing more than eight hours per day. Most protection was seen in those taking between one to seven hours activity per day. These data suggested that too much activity could have a deleterious effect on heart disease rates. This 'inverted U hypothesis' (figure 4.1) suggests that *more* is not necessarily better, and that there is a threshold above which the effects of exercise may be damaging. We shall return to this concept later.

Brunner, and Manelis (1960) – the Israeli Kibbutzim Study

The *Lancet* of November 1960 published an article by D. Brunner and G. Manelis on the incidence of ischaemic heart disease among members of communal settlements (kibbutzim) in Israel. There are obvious advantages in an epidemiological study of this sort, since the members of such communal settlements are ethnically homogeneous and the environmental conditions, such as housing, diet, recreation, cultural activity, are virtually uniform. In this way, many factors that would tend to distort studies of other populations are effectively removed. Social status is the same for everyone in the kibbutzim, irrespective of whether the individual is a teacher, clerk, doctor or manual worker.

The survey examined the incidence of heart disease over the decade from 1949 to 1959 in 8,500 people living in a total of 58 different settlements. There is a comprehensive medical service in the kibbutzim and medical information was, therefore, readily available. In the ten-year period, there occurred 111 cases of heart attack; 34 patients died and 77 survived. Of the 4,000 women, only nine suffered a heart attack; of these two died and seven survived. In the communal settlements approximately 30 per cent of those studied were engaged in sedentary work. The results showed that for non-sedentary male workers (i.e., physically active), the annual incidence of heart disease was 1.36 per 1,000 whereas for sedentary males the annual incidence was 4.1 per 1,000. In other words, the sedentary group had three times more heart disease than the non-sedentary group. These results thus supported the conclusions of Morris' original study, which suggested that exercise exerted a protective role against heart disease.

Taylor and Co-workers (1962) – the American Railroad Study

In 1962 another study from America was published in the *American Journal of Public Health*. Taylor and others at the University of Minnesota School of Public Health analysed the health records of almost 200,000 men working in the American railroad industry. Again, the evidence showed that those workers involved in sedentary occupations, such as the ticket collectors, suffered more heart disease than their physically active colleagues, who were involved in more manual occupations within the industry.

This study, as with most other epidemiological studies of this kind, has been criticized on a number of counts, including the accusation that the employees of the railroad industry are not typical of the general population. This charge cannot, of course, be completely refuted, but, on the other hand, we ask the question again, why should employees of the railroad industry be, in essence, any different from the rest of us?

Kahn and Co-workers (1963) – the USA Postal Workers Study

Kahn and his colleagues studied postal workers in the USA, comparing heart attack rates in sedentary groups, such as the sorting clerks, with those in the more physically active groups, such as the postmen. Their findings corresponded essentially with those of Morris and others who, as we have seen, studied postal workers in England. The active mail carriers, i.e., postmen, had a 33–50 per cent lower incidence of heart disease than the sedentary clerks, and they were also less likely to die suddenly from a heart attack.

Hames and McDonough (1965) – the Evans County Study

In 1965, Dr Curtis Hames and his colleagues published the results of an extensive epidemiological study of cardiovascular disease which had been carried out in Evans County, Georgia. This fascinating piece of research stemmed from the essentially simple observation that white people in the area appeared to have a much higher incidence of heart disease than blacks, despite the fact that the black population had a higher intake of animal fats and also had higher blood pressures.

Evans County is located on the coastal plains, about 60 miles inland from the port city of Savannah, Georgia. The study population consisted of all persons aged 40–74 and a 50 per cent random sample of those aged 15–39 years. Examinations were performed on a total of 3,102 persons and consisted of a full medical history, physical examination, estimation of blood cholesterol, chest X-ray and a 12-lead electrocardiograph. The study was launched in 1960 and reports appeared first in 1965 and then subsequently.

The Evans County Study provided much interesting and valuable data, and in general supported Morris' original hypothesis, i.e., that physical activity provides a measure of protection against heart disease. In essence, the study confirmed that there was a substantial difference in the incidence of heart disease between the black and white populations, with the white males suffering approximately three times more heart disease than the blacks. Moreover, this difference could not be accounted for in terms of other conventional coronary risk factors, such as blood pressure, cigarette smoking or blood cholesterol levels.

It was social class which accounted for the differences, with the higher social classes (predominantly whites) having the higher incidence of heart disease. The social class differences, in turn, could be accounted for in terms of occupation. The basic economy of Evans County was related to agriculture, and most of the lower class workers, involved in essentially manual occupations such as sharecropping and other labouring jobs, were black. The white population was composed of farm owners and other managerial and professional groups, who clearly have a much more sedentary lifestyle. The essential difference between the groups, therefore, lay in the amount of physical activity performed during working hours, with the poorer, lower social class blacks having a high level of physical activity and a correspondingly low incidence of heart disease, while the more sedentary white population, comprising the higher social class groups, had a high incidence of heart disease. Racial factors could not account for the differences because lower social class whites employed in manual occupations shared a low incidence of heart disease with their black fellow-workers.

During the course of this study, the physical activity/heart disease association was explored further with additional data being collected on one occupational type – the farm owners. It was observed that owners of small farms performed more physically demanding work than owners of large farms. The main reasons for these differences lay in the fact that less mechanization and less hired help was available on the smaller farms. If physical activity was in some way related to heart disease, and if physical activity was related to farm size, it should have followed that there was a relationship between the number of acres farmed and the incidence of heart disease. When the results were analysed, it was found that such a relationship did indeed exist, with owners of large farms (189–10,750 acres) having approximately three times the incidence of heart disease compared with the small farm owners (20–188 acres).

One or two points arising from this study merit special attention. The authors point out, quite correctly, that the argument that the genetic make-up of the individual concerned determined his heart attack risk could not explain the differences in heart attack rates between the various groups. If certain individuals do have a particular predisposition to develop heart disease, then why should they form themselves into convenient groups, apparently being only limited to certain social classes? Furthermore, if such a genetic predisposition were accounted for in terms of racial differences, it could not account for the differences in heart attack rates among whites in different occupations.

The only way in which genetic factors could explain the differences between the groups would be for the genetically less susceptible individuals to have somehow self-selected themselves into the labouring occupations. This theory stretches credibility to breaking point, since for most negroes the concept of occupational selection would not be one with which they were familiar. Most would be pleased to take any reasonable occupation available – there would hardly be very much choice in the matter.

In summary, therefore, the Evans County study demonstrated a clear association between activity patterns and coronary heart disease, and furthermore showed that it acted as an entirely independent risk factor. It was interesting to note that the increasing industrialization of Evans County during the 1960s brought substantial changes in the occupational profile of the population. As the area became more affluent, the poorer whites who had hitherto worked in manual occupations moved up the socio-economic scale and subsequently developed a high incidence of heart disease. Only those who did not achieve such affluence and continued in their manual occupations remained relatively resistant to heart disease.

Shapiro and Weinblatt (1969) – the New York Health Insurance Plan Study

In 1969 an analysis of approximately 110,000 adults enrolled in the Health Insurance Plan of Greater New York was published by Shapiro and his colleagues. The members of the plan were categorized according to their levels of physical activity, and it was found that the least active group had twice the risk of suffering a heart attack compared with the more active group (8.5 per 1,000 and 4.2 per 1,000 respectively). Not only was the incidence of heart disease much higher in those with sedentary occupations, but they were also twice as likely to die from a heart attack when it occurred (48 per cent death rate in the sedentary group as compared with 22 per cent in the active). Interestingly, the major differences in heart attack incidence were between the sedentary and the moderately active groups, with little additional benefit being found in those classified as vigorously active. This tends to support the work of Zukel and others (see above), which showed that *more* exercise was not necessarily better.

The Shapiro study has been criticized for being incomplete in several respects, e.g., the fact that other coronary risk factors were not taken into account, and also that the number of patients who were actually examined in detail was relatively small (156 out of a sample of 110,000). The authors were themselves cautious about the interpretation of their findings, but the suggestion that physical exercise may exert a beneficial effect was still very apparent, and was certainly as good an explanation of the data as any other offered.

Morris (1973) – the British Civil Servants Study

More than 20 years after his original pioneering study of the London Transport workers, Morris published a further major epidemiological survey in the *Lancet* in February 1973. The title of the paper was 'Vigorous exercise in leisure time and the incidence of coronary heart disease'.

Between 1968 and 1970, 16,882 male executive grade civil servants aged 40–60 years from across Britain recorded their leisure-time physical activity patterns for a Friday and Saturday and completed a questionnaire on habits and personal history. The first report was published in 1973 after a three-year period, and a subsequent longer-term follow-up report was published in December 1980 after some eight and a half years.

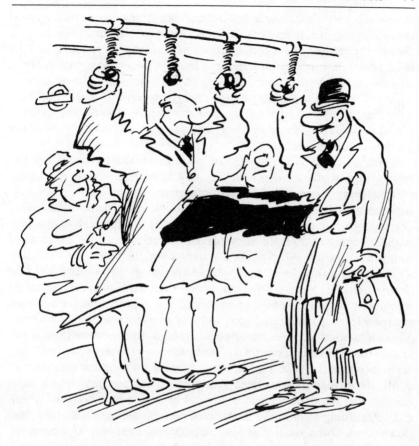

For men engaging in 'vigorous' leisure-time activity during the two sample days, the risk of a fatal heart attack was about 40 per cent that of their colleagues reporting no vigorous exercise, and for non-fatal episodes of coronary heart disease the risk was 50 per cent. In other words, not only did the vigorous exercisers have less heart disease, they were also much less likely to die from it. Those subjects engaged in lighter forms of physical activity showed no significant benefit. It is interesting to note that the beneficial effect of 'vigorous' exercise was seen throughout the age range studied, and especially in late middle-age.

There are a number of important points about this study which merit further attention. First, we should note that Morris opted to study 'leisure-time' activity patterns as opposed to occupational exercise profiles. This is because work in advanced societies has become more sedentary as a result of increasing technology, so any contribution to public health is more likely to be derived from exercise taken in leisure time.

Secondly, we should note that Morris' study showed definite benefit from 'vigorous' exercise. The fact that the word 'vigorous' was used is important, because it suggested a threshold of *intensity* required to produce beneficial cardiovascular effects; no such benefit was seen in those subjects engaged in lighter forms of physical activity. Morris defined 'vigorous' physical activity as a peak energy expenditure of 7.5 kcal/min, equivalent to heavy industrial work. Examples of such activity patterns included running, jogging, cycling, swimming, tennis, walking in rough country, hill climbing etc.

Hitherto it had been shown that patterns of activity had a definite relationship to the incidence of coronary heart disease and the classic exercise/heart disease hypothesis suggested an inverse relationship between the two, i.e., the more the physical activity, the less the risk of developing heart disease. Morris' data changed this hypothesis in a profoundly important way. He suggested that attention should be focused not so much on the *amount* of physical activity as on the *intensity*.

To illustrate this, let us suppose that you are going to spend 100 kcal during exercise. Morris' argument shows that 100 kcal spent during 10 minutes of vigorous running or swimming has a quite different effect on the body from spending that same 100 kcal during 30 minutes of walking. Vigorous activity involves major muscle groups, utilizes more than 50 per cent of the subject's maximum oxygen uptake (see chapter 6) and substantially increases the heart rate and therefore the total cardiac output.

Morris further demonstrated that a specific time spent on vigorous exercise was required before the physical exercise would become 'beneficial'. According to him, the duration of exercise required was more than 30 minutes, and a total of at least one hour of such activity during the Friday/Saturday period appeared to be advantageous.

Thus, while demonstrating once again the beneficial effects of exercise, Morris' work showed that certain requirements in terms of exercise duration and intensity must be fulfilled before such benefits are forthcoming. Assuming that these requirements are met, however, 'The generality of the advantage', to quote Morris 'suggests that vigorous exercise is a natural defence of the body, with a protective effect on the ageing heart against ischaemia and its consequences'.

Paffenbarger and Hale (1975) – the San Francisco Dock Workers Study

In order to assess the role of physical exercise in reducing heart disease mortality in San Francisco longshoremen (dock workers), Paffenbarger and Hale followed a total of 6,351 subjects for a period of 22 years (1951–1972). During this period, these subjects (aged 35–74 years) contributed 92,645 man-years of work, of which 27,667 constituted heavy work (5.2–7.5 kcal/min), 21,456 moderate work (2.4–5.0) and 43,522 light work (1.5–2.0).

On average, those jobs classified as 'heavy' required 1,876 kcal above the normal daily requirement, moderate 1,473 kcal, and light only 865 kcal more per day.

During the follow-up period, 598 longshoremen died from coronary heart disease. Of this total number of deaths, 66 occurred in the heavy work group, 107 in the moderate and 425 in the light. Taking into account the age-specific and age-adjusted death rates, there was an 80 per cent risk of fatal coronary disease incurred by the sedentary workers as compared with the more vigorous longshoremen. This differential in terms of heart disease incidence persisted even when the effect of other conventional risk factors, such as cigarette smoking and blood pressure, was taken into account. In other words, exercise was shown to be an entirely independent risk factor.

Finally, Paffenbarger once again demonstrated a minimum 'threshold' for exercise intensity (5.2–7.5 kcal/min), before the beneficial effects of physical activity were observed. It was in the high activity group that the real benefit was observed (relative risk of heart disease 1.0), with the moderate and light activity subjects showing no significant benefit (relative risk at 1.7 and 1.8, respectively).

In summary, therefore, these data suggested that 'vigorous physical exercise, as defined by an apparent threshold or critical level of energy output, is associated with reduced risk of coronary mortality, particularly sudden death'.

Paffenbarger, Wing, and Hyde (1978) – the Harvard University Alumni Study

Following on from their study of the San Francisco longshoremen, Paffenbarger and his co-workers examined the relationship between physical activity and heart disease in 16,936 Harvard University male alumni (old boys), aged 35–74 years. The subjects were classified by hours per week of light or strenuous sport, and by their equivalent energy output in kilocalories per week. Analysis of the data indicated that high level energy expenditure was protective against both fatal and non-fatal coronary disease. There was, in fact, a 64 per cent greater incidence of heart attacks in those with sedentary recreational habits as compared with those who took vigorous exercise. The benefit existed at all age levels between 35 and 74 years, and this study once again confirmed a threshold of exercise intensity, below which no improvement in the incidence of heart disease was demonstrable.

Two further points deserve mention. First, the study showed clearly that the beneficial effects of exercise cannot be stored on a long-term basis. Those subjects who were physically active as students but who subsequently became sedentary, showed no reduction in heart attack risk. Benefit was only demonstrable for those who were able to maintain a physically active lifestyle on leaving university. In other words, you cannot put a lot of physical activity into the 'bank' in the early years and expect that this will provide some benefit in later years. Secondly, the study also demonstrated an *upper* threshold for physical activity (2,000–2,500 kcal/week) above which no additional benefit in terms of reduced risk for heart disease was observed. In other words, running 100 miles a week probably does no more good than running 20 miles a week.

Garcia-Palmieri and Co-workers (1982) – the Puerto Rico Heart Program Study

A study by Palmieri and his colleagues of 2,585 rural and 6,208 urban men aged 45–64 years participating in the Puerto Rico Heart Program was reported in the *American Journal of Cardiology* in 1982. This prospective epidemiological study was initiated in 1965 and the subjects were followed-up for a period of just over eight years. The incidence of coronary disease and the prevalence of conventional risk factors was assessed.

An index of physical activity was derived from each individual history, and rural men were found to have higher mean levels of overall activity as well as higher levels of heavy activity than the urban men. When activity patterns were then related to the incidence of heart disease, it was found that the highest incidence of disease was related to the lowest levels of physical activity. Thus, once again, this prospective investigation supports the conclusions of previous studies, that increased physical activity may protect against coronary heart disease.

Pomrehn and Wallace (1984) – the Iowa Farmers Study

This study of heart disease mortality in Iowa farmers was reported in the *Journal of the American Medical Association*. Pomrehn and his co-workers analysed 62,000 deaths in men aged 20–64 years, between 1964 and 1978. Death rates were compared between farming and non-farming occupations, and cardiovascular risk factors between groups were also examined in detail.

Farmers smoked less frequently (19 v. 44 per cent) and engaged in exercise more frequently (83 v. 40 per cent) than non-farmers. Treadmill performance in farm men confirmed a higher level of physical fitness than that found in the non-farmers.

In summary, the study showed that Iowa farmers had significantly lower death rates from heart disease than other Iowa men, and that lifestyle accounted for a significant portion of this mortality advantage. Both the total mortality and the mortality from heart disease reflected the healthy behaviour patterns of farm people, in that they smoked far less and took more physical exercise than their non-farming counterparts.

Thus, more than 30 years since Morris' original report, evidence continues to accumulate in support of the general hypothesis that high levels of physical activity are related to a low incidence of coronary heart disease.

We have reviewed a number of studies showing a definite relationship between activity patterns and heart disease and, although the analysis is neither detailed nor comprehensive, we do believe that it represents a fair cross-section of the evidence available. All these studies show definite benefit from regular vigorous exercise, and most have been criticized to varying degrees for defects in data collection, study design and methodology.

But what about the other side of the coin? Are there any studies showing no benefit from exercise in terms of reduced risk for coronary heart disease? There are indeed, although they are relatively few in number and, as with all the other studies, they also have deficiencies in design and construction.

Malhotra (1967) – the Indian Railway Workers Study

In the *British Heart Journal* of 1967, Malhotra published a study called 'Epidemiology of ischaemic heart disease in India with special reference to causation'. The study related to 1.15 million railway workers between the ages of 18 and 55 years, serving on the eight zonal railways in different parts of India. The period of study was from 1 January 1958 to 31 December 1962. By analysing the various medical and hospital records and death certificates, a pattern of morbidity and mortality from heart disease for each of the eight railway zones could be established.

In essence, the study showed that although there were major geographical differences with regard to the incidence of heart disease, there was no evidence to suggest that physical activity, cigarette smoking, diet or stress could account for the observed variations; i.e., physical activity *per se* did not appear to exert any beneficial effect. Indeed, of the activity grades examined (clerks, fitters and sweepers), the fitters and sweepers, which were regarded as the more active grades, actually had a higher incidence of heart disease than did the clerks, who were classified as sedentary.

This evidence is clearly contrary to the conclusions of the other major studies which we have examined, but there are a number of points upon which this study can justifiably be criticized. First, although the author claims that physical activity, 'stress' and cigarette smoking appeared to make no contribution to the incidence of heart disease among workers in the various railways zones, it must be said that the data obtained on these parameters were at best highly questionable, and at worst worthless.

'Stress' for example, was assessed by considering the number of disciplinary actions against each individual for lapses in job performance. This is hardly a comprehensive means of assessing individual sources of stress. The term itself is not amenable to precise definition, and to use such arbitrary criteria for its assessment is dubious. In addition, even this meagre information was incomplete because some of the railway zones did not provide any information concerning 'stress' ratings for individuals employed in their region.

The evidence regarding cigarette smoking is just as questionable. Data on smoking were not based upon individual smoking habits, but rather upon total cigarette sales in each region obtained from trade sources. It is not known what percentage of sales in each region could be accounted for by railway workers. In other words, this information simply reflects regional smoking habits and says nothing about the smoking habits of individual railway employees. Since so little is known about individual smoking habits, it cannot be claimed that smoking was not a significant risk factor. There is simply no evidence to support such a conclusion.

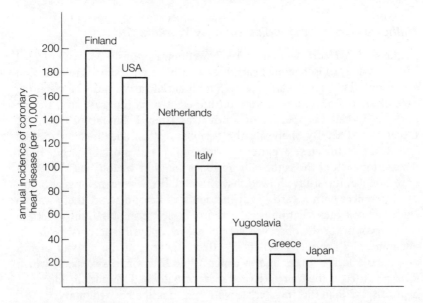

Figure 4.2   Incidence of coronary heart disease in the 'Seven Nations Study'.

Finally, the claim that physical activity patterns were not important also deserves further examination. The supposed differences in activity patterns between clerks, fitters and sweepers were not accurately quantified. We are told only that the sweepers and fitters were physically active and that the clerks were sedentary. The difference in calorific expenditure between groups was not examined and we cannot tell whether their various energy classifications would be regarded as moderately or vigorously active. Perhaps the energy gradients between these working groups were not sufficient to produce any observable differences in the incidence of heart disease. In other words, perhaps the fitters and sweepers were not sufficiently active to obtain benefit, and this may reflect cultural, geographical and climatic variations.

In summary, therefore, it is clear that the evidence concerning the role of physical activity, cigarette smoking and 'stress' in this study is highly questionable. We can hardly accept the author's conclusion that these factors made no significant contribution to the incidence of heart disease in the population studied, and in particular the role of physical activity is not quantifiable.

Keys (1970) – the 'Seven Nations Study'

An international cooperative study on the epidemiology of heart disease was reported by Keys in 1970. The 'Seven Nations Study', as it came to be known, reported data on 12,770 men aged 40–59 years in Finland, Japan, Italy, The Netherlands, Yugoslavia, Greece and the USA. The study of the individuals taking part was carefully standardized throughout the seven countries and the examination procedures included questionnaires on work, family history and previous medical history. Detailed physical examination was performed and the investigations also included a simplified exercise stress test. In addition, there were frequent changes of professional personnel between national teams in order to remove any obvious medical bias when performing the assessments. After the baseline evaluations had been made, the sample population was followed closely and a complete reassessment was carried out again after five years.

There were major differences in the incidence of coronary heart disease in each of the seven countries during the five-year period studied, with the USA and Finland showing the highest incidence, and Japan, Greece and Yugoslavia being on the low side (figure 4.2).

When the data were examined in terms of conventional coronary risk factors, it was clear that cigarette smoking, obesity and physical activity patterns bore no clearly defined relationship to the incidence of heart disease in the seven countries observed. For example, although 60 per cent of men in the USA were classified as sedentary compared with only 10 per cent in Finland, the Finns nevertheless had a higher incidence of disease than the Americans. Also, although 59 per cent of Japanese men smoked more than ten cigarettes a day (more heavy smokers than any other country), Japanese men still had the lowest incidence of heart disease of all the nations studied.

The closest correlation with the observed incidence of disease was found with blood pressure levels and levels of blood cholesterol. The latter was in turn related to the proportion of calories in the diet derived from animal fats.

In summary, the 'Seven Nations Study' showed substantial differences in the incidence of heart disease throughout the seven countries, differences that appeared to bear no relationship to physical activity, obesity or cigarette smoking. The only factors that could account for the international variations in disease incidence were cholesterol and blood pressure levels.

On balance, this was obviously a well-constructed study. Although it showed no clearly defined benefit from physical activity, it was not entirely negative in its findings. The evidence from the USA sample, made up of 2,571 employees of the railroad industry, did show that the incidence of heart disease in men engaged in sedentary occupations was in fact 16 per cent higher than that observed in the physically more active switchmen. The difference was not statistically significant, but we believe (as Keys himself stated) that the sample size may have been too small for any clear association to be defined.

Thus, although at first sight the study appears to contradict the conclusions of the other studies we have examined, the sample size in each country may not have been sufficient to produce statistically significant correlations.

Chapman and Co-workers (1957) – the Los Angeles Civil Servants Study

Chapman and his colleagues studied a population of 2,252 Los Angeles civil servants for a period of two to three years. This study actually reported a greater incidence of death from coronary heart disease in the physically active groups as compared with those having the lowest levels of physical activity, by a factor of about 25 per cent. Like most other studies, this too could be criticized on various points; in this case perhaps the most obvious would be that the sample size was relatively small. For example, Morris' study of civil servants was made up of a sample of almost 17,000 more than seven times larger than the sample studied by Chapman.

Weighing the Evidence

All the studies which we have examined (and they represent only part of the mass of data available) are imperfect in one way or another. The perfect epidemiological study has never been performed, but this is in the nature of the subject matter under investigation. As we said before, all science is probability, and nowhere is this more true than in the study of medicine and related disciplines. Bearing these points in mind, it is perhaps worthwhile examining some of the more important criticisms levelled against the evidence supporting the case for exercise.

The particular group in question is not representative of the population as a whole

This is always a perfectly valid criticism and can be applied to virtually every population ever studied. Thus, it can be argued that Morris' London Transport workers are not typical of the population as a whole, and that therefore we cannot draw any broad conclusions about the protective role of exercise. The same argument will be levelled against postal workers and civil servants, again claiming that what is true for them does not apply to the rest of us. This argument will equally have to apply to the dock workers in San Fancisco, ex-Harvard alumni, farmers in Iowa, people enrolled in the health insurance plan of New York etc. etc. It follows from this argument that each of these groups must be endowed with a specific and unique constitutional and genetic background, which makes them quite distinct from the rest of us. However, the more data obtained on ever-more diverse groups of workers, dimishes the credibility of the argument. No doubt the study groups do differ in some respects, but that is not at issue. The real question is whether the differences are so profound as to account for the major differences observed in the incidence of heart disease.

The problem with this argument is that it lacks common sense. After all, why should postal workers, railwaymen, dock workers or civil servants be in any real sense different from the rest of us? What evidence is there to suggest that these supposed differences, making them so atypical of the rest of us, actually exist? In reality, there is no evidence at all. The criticism can only ever be rejected completely, however, when every occupational group has been studied and the accumulated evidence continues to show benefit from exercise. Clearly, this will never happen, and so the argument, from a purely logical and scientific point of view, is irrefutable. There is, nevertheless, not the slightest reason for believing it to be true.

Genetic and constitutional factors account for 'self-selection' into particular occupations, and also for the degree of resistance or susceptibility to heart disease

This argument is really an extension of the previous one, and suggests that the reason why one particular group under study is not typical of the remainder of the population is that they have specific genetic and constitutional factors which make them different. For example, in Morris' original study of transport workers, it might be argued that bus drivers were somehow genetically programmed to choose that particular form of occupation and, at the same time, they have inherited a high degree of susceptibility to heart disease. The conductors, on the other hand, were a group who self-selected for a job with higher levels of physical activity, but who coincidentially inherited a certain degree of protection from heart disease. The difference in activity patterns was therefore purely coincidental, and has nothing to do with protection from coronary heart disease. Thus, runs this argument, irrespective of how much exercise you do, it is genetic factors which determine the occupation that is chosen, and also the degree of resistance or susceptibility to heart disease.

There are a number of problems with this argument. First, the idea that 'self-selection' determines occupational activity is hard to accept. Negroes in Evans County or lower social classes in Puerto Rico probably have very little choice as to which occupational activity they assume. 'Self-selection' implies a flexibility of choice which often does not exist.

Even if we are prepared to accept that constitutional factors predispose us to choosing particular jobs, however, it is hard to accept that the gene responsible for the relative degree of susceptibility should distribute itself in such a non-random way. If such a genetic factor existed, it would surely distribute itself evenly among all social groups and occupational activities. For example, in the Evans County study it was found that higher social class whites had a much greater incidence of heart disease than lower social class blacks and whites, and social class was clearly related to occupational activity. If the genetic argument were true, we would have to accept that constitutional factors not only determined which social class and occupational activity an individual would adopt, but also his resistance to heart disease. This seems to be stretching credibility again, and it would not explain how those whites in a lower social class and manual occupation, who presumably have a genetic resistance to heart disease, should lose that resistance when they become more affluent and move up the socioeconomic scale. One would have to postulate that the gene controlling resistance to heart disease expresses itself according to the income of the individual concerned.

Furthermore, in Paffenbarger's study of Harvard alumni, those individuals who had chosen vigorous activities while at university only gained benefit in later life if they maintained high levels of physical activity. Academics who had been sedentary while at university but who took up vigorous exercise in later life did gain benefit in terms of reduced incidence of heart disease. If the 'pre-selection' theory – that individuals who are genetically endowed with healthy hearts choose more active pursuits – were true, then one would not have expected to see benefit in the more sedentary academic groups who took up exercise in later life. One would have to postulate that the gene controlling activity patterns and resistance to heart disease, only began to express itself in later years. In the groups who exercised at university, but then became sedentary in later life, one would have to postulate the converse, i.e., that they were genetically programmed to have healthy hearts and high levels of physical activity only in the early part of their lives, but later this genetic influence somehow failed to express itself. This intermittent expression of such constitutional influences hardly seems likely.

There is no absolutely irrefutable proof that exercise exerts a protective effect against coronary heart disease

This criticism is completely justified, but is not peculiar to the exercise/ heart disease hypothesis. A great many principles that underlie the practice of modern medicine are not amenable to absolute proof but we are content, in most cases, to accept the probability of the evidence. For example, there is no absolutely conclusive proof that cigarette smoking causes lung cancer, but there is as near to a cause and effect relationship as one is ever likely to see. If we were to wait until such 'proof' were available, a great many people would die very unpleasant and unnecessary deaths during the period of our equivocation.

The evidence suggesting that high animal fat intakes are related to coronary heart disease is far from conclusive, but there is sufficient evidence available at present for several very distinguished bodies to recommend that the population in general should substantially reduce its intake of animal fats. At the very least, there is no real evidence that such a reduction in fat intake would do us any *harm*, and so recommending such dietary modifications would certainly seem prudent.

There are countless areas in medicine where absolute proof is lacking, but where recommendations for treatment have to be based upon available evidence. In this respect, the heart disease/exercise hypothesis is no different. The reader should bear in mind that no study has ever been published which showed acceleration of atheroma ('furring-up' of the arteries) in humans as a result of exercise. There is a great deal of evidence to suggest that exercise exerts a powerfully protective effect, and so for this reason, it would seem prudent to recommend increasing the general activity patterns of the population.

Conclusions

We have examined some of the criticisms that are often levelled against the case for exercise. The concept of pre-selection, which we have already discussed, is one of the most common. The claim is that protection against heart disease is under genetic control and is therefore something over which we can have no influence. It is also claimed that this genetic protection tends to make such individuals more physically able than the rest of us, and therefore more likely to engage in vigorous exercise. In other words, it is not exercise that offers you protection against heart disease, but simply that you were genetically less likely to get it in the first place.

There are a number of problems with this which we have already discussed, but it is highly improbable that this 'pre-selection' can account for all of the differences in heart disease incidence which we observe between groups with varying levels of physical activity. The claim that those who exercise are genetically programmed to do so and therefore have a higher physical capacity than the remainder of the population, is simply not true.

Some people appear to claim that exercise is the panacea for all our ills. This is a naïve and simplistic viewpoint which the informed reader will obviously reject. To claim, however, that exercise offers no potential health benefits and that the hypothesis that it does so is nothing more than a 'myth', is a grotesque and dangerous distortion of the truth. There is ample evidence that exercise has an important part to play in disease prevention, and while the data are not conclusive, they are certainly compelling.

This is not to say that we all have to become marathon runners; it is rather to suggest that we should reclassify the population as active as opposed to sedentary. Those of us who live in the real world in which large numbers of people die from cardiac disease, many of them needlessly, cannot allow ourselves the luxury of sitting back until a causal association between exercise and reduction in heart disease has been established. We have to take a more pragmatic approach, and ask ourselves this question: Would advocating increased levels of physical activity in the population as a whole bring about a substantial improvement in public health, an improvement which far outweighs any potential harmful effect? In the authors' opinion, the answer is unequivocally 'Yes'.

5

The Effects of Exercise

The mechanisms by which exercise is believed to reduce the risk of heart disease are not know with certainty, and probably comprise a number of separate, although related, factors. This chapter will consider some of these factors.

Improved Cardiovascular Efficiency

We have seen in chapter 2 that the oxygen supply to the heart is obtained from blood flowing through the arteries. It follows that when the arteries are blocked, a potential imbalance occurs between the oxygen requirements of the heart, and the amount of blood which the arteries are able to supply. When such an imbalance is present, the heart becomes starved of oxygen, a situation referred to in medical terminology as 'ischaemia'. This situation is potentially serious, and means that the heart muscle is endangered.

The oxygen requirements of the heart can be roughly estimated by the 'rate–pressure product', i.e.,

cardiac oxygen requirement = heart rate × systolic blood pressure

For example, the rate-pressure product at a heart rate of 190 beats per minute and a systolic blood pressure of 220 mmHg (typical values at maximum exercise) would be

$$220 \times 190 = 41,800$$

Clearly, if we can reduce the heart rate or the systolic blood pressure at any given workload, then the oxygen requirement of the heart at that point will be less. This means that in a situation where the blood supply to the heart is potentially limited, the relative threat to the heart of being deprived of oxygen is much less. For example, if the heart rate were reduced to 170 in the above equation, the rate–pressure product would be as follows

$$220 \times 170 = 37,400$$

Thus, reducing the heart rate by 20 beats at any given workload, may produce a substantial reduction of oxygen requirement for the heart (in the above case, by more than ten per cent). Because an imbalance between supply and demand of oxygen is less likely to occur, the health of the heart is much more assured.

One of the effects of sustained exercise training is to bring about a reduction in heart rates for sub-maximal workloads. This means that the oxygen requirements of the heart are much less and the heart is able to function safely and efficiently.

Even in patients with established coronary artery disease, aerobic training produces many of the same cardiovascular adaptations that occur in normal people. Indeed, many patients who suffer with angina (chest pain due to lack of oxygen to the heart) are able to raise the threshold at which they develop pain by using controlled aerobic training. Since the oxygen requirements of the heart at each given workload are less, these subjects are able to do proportionately more exercise before the pain occurs. In some cases they are even able to dispense with medication.

Aerobic training may reduce the resting heart rate very substantially. In our own laboratory it is by no means unusual to see well-trained 'elite' athletes with resting heart rates of only 38 beats per minute. This is approximately half the rate of a normal, untrained individual (72). Clearly, at rest the oxygen requirements for the trained as compared with the untrained individual are very different. If we assume a blood pressure of 120 mmHg for each, then the approximate oxygen demands in each case are 4,560 and 8,640 (for the athelete and untrained individual respectively). It is easy to see, therefore, how the trained heart is much more efficient in delivering blood to the tissues and requires much less oxygen than the heart of the sedentary individual.

If the heart of the athlete can achieve as much in 38 contractions as the ordinary individual does in 72 beats, then clearly the athlete's heart must be pumping more blood per contraction. Athletes do indeed have a substantially increased 'stroke volume' (the amount of blood ejected from the heart during each contraction) when compared with untrained individuals. The sedentary individual during exercise will eject approximately 120 ml per contraction, and the total cardiac output per minute is 120 ×

heart rate. If we assume a maximum heart rate during exercise of 200 beats/min, then the total cardiac output is 200×120 ml = 24,000 ml or 24 l/min. At rest, the stroke volume may be about 80 ml with a heart rate of 72 beats/min, giving a resting cardiac output of 72×80 = 5,760 ml or 5.8 l/min.

During exercise, therefore, the cardiac output may increase to four or five times the resting level. In the trained athlete, the stroke volume during exercise may be 180 ml or even higher, and if we again assume a maximum heart rate of 200 beats/min, the cardiac output is 200×180 = 36,000 ml or 36 l/min. At rest, the stroke volume may be 100 ml with a heart rate of perhaps 45 beats/min, giving a cardiac output of 4,500 ml or 4.5 l/min. This means that the trained athlete may increase his cardiac output during exercise to six, seven or even eight times the resting level.

The increase in stroke volume and, therefore, of cardiac output, is brought about by changes in the heart muscle. As a result of endurance training the heart increases in size (a process known as hypertrophy), and also contracts more efficiently. In addition, the volume of the chambers in the heart also increases, with the capacity of the left ventricles in trained individuals being up to 35 per cent greater than in sedentary subjects. There is a clear correlation between the size of the heart and the maximum cardiac output.

Finally, regular aerobic training may help to increase the electrical stability of the heart and prevent dangerous disturbances in cardiac rhythm. We shall see later that certain types of rhythm disturbance during exercise may be potentially life-threatening and anything which helps to reduce the likelihood of such events must be beneficial. The evidence for increased electrical stability in humans is inconclusive, but Billman and co-workers have demonstrated a reduction in life-threatening disturbances in rhythm in dogs who were given programmes of exercise training.

In summary, the beneficial cardiovascular effects of exercise training are related to an increase in heart size, a more efficient heart muscle (myocardium) with a reduced oxygen demand at rest and during exercise, and perhaps a more electrically stable heart with a reduced likelihood of life-threatening rhythm disturbances.

Direct Effects on Coronary Arteries

Aerobic training appears to improve myocardial blood flow and consequently the oxygen supply to the heart. Evidence from post-mortem studies in great endurance athletes has demonstrated main coronary arteries with diameters up to three times their usual width – although whether this is an effect of exercise *per se* or merely an accident of birth is not proven. There is also evidence that exercise not only increases the diameter of the coronary arteries and therefore the myocardial blood flow, but also substantially reduces the development of atheroma. Thus, the arteries are not only larger, but also have much less blockage due to the 'furring-up' process. Studies showing such reductions in the development of atheroma are lacking in human beings because of the difficulty in evaluating the state of the coronary arteries at regular intervals and other technical and ethical problems. However, there is good evidence from animal models that exercise does protect against the formation of atheroma.

Kramsch and his colleagues, at the Boston University Medical Center, published a fascinating study assessing the effect of exercise training on the progress of atheroma in the coronary arteries of monkeys. This particular group of primates is generally thought to provide a good model for the investigation of such disease. In essence, the study involved 27 young adult male *Macaca fascicularis* monkeys from Malaysia. They were randomly divided into three groups of nine animals each, and then studied for a period of 36 months. One group was fed a diet high in saturated fats and likely to produce atheroma in the coronary arteries (an atherogenic diet.) This group remained entirely sedentary. The second group was also fed a high fat diet, but in this case they were also given controlled exercise on a treadmill for a period of 18 months. The third group, which acted as a control, was fed a normal diet and also remained sedentary.

At post-mortem, the differences between the monkeys who exercised on the high fat diet and those who took the high fat diet but did not exercise were striking. The exercising monkeys had very much less atheroma in their coronary arteries and also had arteries that were substantially wider than in the non-exercising group.

It is interesting that the level of exercise in the conditioned monkeys was comparable to jogging in human beings. The study provides direct evidence that even in the presence of a high fat diet likely to produce large amounts of atheroma, exercise can exert a powerful protective effect. In those monkeys who remained sedentary on the atherogenic diet, the diet induced easily visible coronary atherosclerosis at post-mortem. In marked contrast, all exercise-conditioned monkeys had coronary arteries that were strikingly wider than even the normal arteries of the sedentary animals, and had no obvious areas of narrowing. This is powerful evidence supporting the case for exercise, and in the authors' own words 'provides direct evidence that long-term regular exercise, even at moderate levels, may be capable of retarding atherosclerotic coronary heart disease in primates'.

In addition, there is also some evidence that exercise may improve 'collateral' blood flow to the heart. In 1957 Eckstein published an interesting study on dogs in which he examined the effects of tying off a branch of the coronary arterial tree so as to induce a non-fatal heart attack. The area of heart muscle supplied by the tied artery was deprived of oxygen and died. The dogs could therefore be considered as post-coronary (i.e. having suffered a coronary thrombosis). The dogs were then divided into two groups – one entirely sedentary and the other exercised regularly. Further evaluation later confirmed that the exercising dogs had developed new coronary vessels which grew around the blocked vessels and eventually made up for the lack of blood supply. These new vessels are referred to in medical terms as 'collaterals'. The sedentary dogs showed no significant evidence of collateral flow.

The evidence for improved collateral flow as a result of exercise in humans, however, is by no means conclusive. Some studies have not been able to demonstrate any improvement in myocardial blood flow as a result of collateral formation. However, improvements in collateral flow may in fact occur through extremely small blood vessels, by what is termed the micro-circulation. If this is the case, then present techniques for assessing coronary flow may be too crude to identify collateral formation.

Although the evidence is somewhat lacking, it seems that improvement in collateral flow does represent a possible mechanism by which exercise may increase myocardial blood flow.

Changes in Blood Pressure

It was pointed out in chapter 3 that elevated blood pressure is generally accepted as one of the major conventional coronary risk factors. There is some evidence that exercise may be beneficial by lowering the blood pressure level in certain subjects. Cooper's studies of more than 3,000 men showed that the resting systolic and diastolic blood pressures were significantly lower in physically fit persons than in those who were in a comparatively poor condition. There is also some evidence that those who have elevated blood pressures at the commencement of an exercise programme may significantly reduce these pressures after a period of aerobic training.

There seems little doubt that in certain individuals useful and even therapeutic reductions in blood pressure may occur as a result of endurance training. However, this may partly be accounted for by a reduction in body fat which results from regular exercise, although no doubt other mechanisms have a part to play. In our own experience the response of blood pressure to exercise training varies somewhat from individual to individual. Hellerstein and his colleagues point out the importance of taking initial blood pressure readings before exercise training commences. In a subject with a low or normal blood pressure prior to training, regular exercise appeared to have little effect on resting blood pressure. If blood pressure was elevated to start with, however, then significant reductions in resting blood pressure (systolic and diastolic) occurred as a result of aerobic conditioning. For certain individuals, therefore, exercise may make a significant contribution to reducing elevated blood pressure levels.

Changes in Blood Lipids (Fats)

The importance of blood fats in the development of coronary disease, and in particular the role of cholesterol and high density lipoprotein (HDL), was discussed in chapter 3 (see also appendix 1). In essence, we regard cholesterol as being of great importance in the development of atheroma, whereas HDL appears to exert a protective effect against the development of atheromatous plaques in the coronary arteries. Therefore, in simple terms, we would tend to regard anything that could reduce cholesterol and increase HDL as having a potentially beneficial effect.

Exercise has very little effect on total serum cholesterol, although it does reduce triglyceride levels (see glossary and appendix 1). There is evidence, however, that exercise does exert a beneficial effect on blood lipids, by increasing levels of HDL which are though to be cardio-protective. Many studies show a clear relationship between levels of HDL and activity patterns within the groups being studied. In one study comparing HDL levels in lumberjacks and electricians, the lumberjacks, whose occupation is obviously very active, had significantly higher levels of HDL than the more inactive electricians. Furthermore, many of the studies show that the type of exercise appears to be important for a rise in HDL to occur. For example, ice hockey players and sprinters, who are not endurance trained, had significantly lower HDL levels than did aerobically trained long-distance runners, and in one study the number of miles run per week was found to be the best predictor of HDL levels. However, it appears that significant elevations in HDL levels can be achieved with relatively modest amounts of exercise which would be well within the reach of the vast majority of the population. In one study, 39 sedentary males with an average age of 33 years were studied before and after two months of jogging, walking or running three times per week. Subjects averaged a total of only 5–6 miles per week, nevertheless, levels of HDL increased substantially from 36.9 to 55.5 per cent of the total blood lipoprotein levels.

In another study of medical students who exercised four times per week for a period of seven weeks, the exercise period consisted of jogging, cycling and calisthenics (stretching exercises) for approximately ten minutes each. This relatively modest exercise pattern resulted in an increase in HDL levels of 16 per cent.

One of the difficulties in evaluating the effect of exercise on HDL levels is that, as we have seen, there are a number of factors apart from exercise which may result in changes in HDL levels. Cigarette smoking, obesity, alcohol and other factors have to be taken into account, since all can produce changes in HDL levels. Despite this, there is still good evidence that exercise improves HDL levels, although the hypothesis remains unproved.

HDL is thought to reduce atherosclerosis by facilitating uptake of cholesterol from the arterial wall. Well-controlled long-term studies should help to resolve the question, and more evidence is likely to be forthcoming in the near future. A particular part of the lipoprotein particle, called an 'apoprotein', may have an important part to play in preventing coronary heart disease. These developments provide an important area for research in the future, and may open a new chapter in our understanding of heart disease.

Changes in Blood Coagulation Factors

An increased tendency for the blood to clot (coagulate) may be an important factor in precipitating heart attacks (see chapter 3). There is some evidence that exercise may exert an important effect in reducing the tendency of the blood to coagulate via a number of mechanisms.

Blood clots are broken down within the body by a complicated process involving a number of biochemical reactions, the collective term for which is 'fibrinolysis'. Increased fibrinolysis reduces the tendency of the blood to form stable clots, and this may be an important factor in helping to prevent such clots occurring within the coronary arteries and precipitating a heart attack. There is evidence that exercise substantially increases fibrinolysis, and this may be one important mechanism of prevention and protection.

In addition, there are small particles in human blood called platelets which are very important in blood clot formation. When they collect together (a process known as aggregation) they help to form the initial stage of a clot by 'plugging' the damaged area. Substances that reduce the tendency for platelets to aggregate in this way may help to prevent clot formation. This is the rationale for giving some patients with established coronary heart disease substances such as aspirin which are known to inhibit platelet aggregation.

However, the body itself produces substances that inhibit platelet aggregation, and a group known as the 'prostaglandins' have attracted particular interest. There is evidence that exercise may increase the levels of prostaglandin PGI2, called 'prostacyclin', which is secreted from blood vessels. PGI2 has been shown to inhibit the aggregation of platelets and, since it is increased as a result of exercise, this may be another possible mechanism by which the beneficial effects of physical training are produced. Much more work is required for this mechanism to be clearly defined, but initial results are promising.

Reduction of Obesity

We shall be discussing the question of obesity in more detail in chapter 6, but the reader will already be aware of the vast amount that is written about diet and dieting. A visit to a newsagent will reveal a bewildering array of information on slimming diets, although most of this is not based upon physiological principles and many of these diets are, frankly, nonsense. They usually have as their main attractions that they are quick, easy and 'effective'. They promise rapid and substantial weight loss in 'days', and since we know that at any given time there are literally millions of people in this country trying to lose weight, the potential market is clearly enormous.

Many individuals do show dramatic weight loss over a period of days, but more than 95 per cent will eventually replace the weight again within a very short period of time. In fact, most of the weight loss that occurs by 'crash' dieting is due to a loss of glycogen and water, rather than to any reduction in body fat. The basic equation remains valid: if your body weight is in a state of equilibrium, your intake of energy in calories from

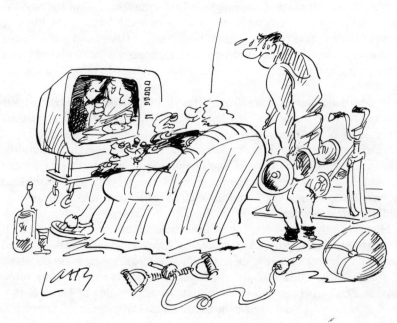

the food you eat must be equal to your energy output. If calorie intake exceeds calorie expenditure, then the excess energy is stored as adipose tissue (i.e., you become fat). If, on the other hand, your expenditure of energy is greater than your intake, you will lose body fat. Clearly, therefore, if you wish to lose weight, you must either reduce your calorie intake, or else increase your energy expenditure. Obesity is very often the result of too little physical activity (i.e. energy expenditure) rather than an excess intake of calories.

There are a number of problems inherent in merely reducing calorie intake as a means of losing body fat. We shall see later that this is often counter-productive (see chapter 6, p. 117).

Exercise has a powerful effect in promoting loss of body fat by bringing about an increase in metabolic rate. A person's metabolic rate is quite simply the rate at which he or she consumes energy. If your metabolic rate is high, you tend to burn large amounts of calories, and this helps to control body fat. Obese people often have low metabolic rates and, therefore, tend to remain fat. Many people have heard the word 'metabolism', and attach some form of mystical quality to it, saying of a fat person, 'It's his metabolism – he can't help it'. The facts, however, are simple: fat people are usually fat because they eat too much, take too little exercise or both. The role of exercise in weight loss has often been neglected, despite the fact that physiologists have known for years that it can have important effects upon metabolic rate and, therefore, upon energy expenditure. Metabolic rate is not fixed and inviolate like the colour of your eyes. It has a dynamic quality and we know that exercise, by increasing the metabolic rate of the body, can burn up a substantial number of calories. By effectively increasing energy output, exercise alone can bring about significant changes in body fat.

In addition, although the body obviously uses many calories during a period of vigorous exercise, it continues to burn calories at a higher rate long after the exercise period has ceased. This is due to the effect of increasing the metabolic rate. The often used argument that running three miles will not burn up many calories and is, therefore, not very effective in controlling body weight, is inaccurate because it fails to take into account the fact that energy expenditure continues at a higher level for many hours after exercise.

Clearly, for many fat people their problem is not so much one of excess food, as of too little exercise. It is very common in our own laboratory to find patients who have been dieting unsuccessfully for many years, despite the fact that they have made genuine reductions for long periods in their overall calorie intake. The prescription of the appropriate form of regular exercise in such cases can often have dramatic and substantial changes in body fat, changes which are real and easy to maintain.

Because obesity is associated with high blood pressure, abnormal blood fats and diabetes, exercise has an indirect but important effect on these factors also. Thus, reducing weight may also mean reducing blood pressure, correcting certain types of blood fat abnormalities and helping in the control of blood sugar levels. We have seen previously that obesity is a significant risk factor for coronary disease, although whether this is because it is often associated with these other abnormalities is not known. What is clear, however, is that by reducing obesity the risk of a heart attack or some other manifestation of coronary heart disease is reduced.

Control of Blood Sugar Levels

Diabetes is a condition in which the level of glucose (sugar) in the blood rises abnormally high because of a reduction in the amount or the effectiveness of insulin. Insulin is a specialized hormone that reduces and controls blood sugar levels within well-defined limits. In diabetics insulin is reduced or defective, and the blood sugar may rise out of control. Apart from the direct dangers of this, diabetics are also known to have a high incidence of complications due to changes in small and large blood vessels supplying a variety of organs within the body. These complications include problems with kidneys and eyes and also the heart, with diabetics having a much higher incidence of coronary heart disease than the remainder of the population. Even in women, the normal pre-menopausal protection from heart disease is lost and they are at even greater risk than men.

It is not absolutely clear why heart disease should be so common in diabetics. Factors that have been suggested include the greater prevalence of hypertension (disputed), obesity and high blood fats, or the occurrence of changes in the blood, e.g., reduced fibrinolysis, increased stickiness of platelets etc. Whatever the determinants may be, it is clearly important to minimize the risk by forbidding smoking, reducing weight, attempting to control abnormal cholesterol levels and ensuring strict control of blood sugar levels.

Exercise has an important part to play in this, because, as we have seen, exercise can facilitate weight loss and changes in blood lipid levels, and may also have an important effect on the platelets and the clotting tendency of the blood. Exercise also has a role to play in the control of blood sugar levels in diabetics, by reducing the insulin demand. The body utilizes glucose during exercise, and the active diabetic requires less insulin than his more sedentary counterpart. The precise mechanism by which this occurs is not well understood, but it is probably associated with a more effective utilization of carbohydrate within the body. Thus, by helping to reduce weight, correcting abnormal blood fat levels and improving glucose tolerance and reducing insulin demand, exercise may have an important potential role in the management of the diabetic.

Control of 'Stress'

Most of us have to live with a certain amount of stress and strain in our everyday lives. We also recognize the need to get away from the everyday worries and pressures from time to time, in order to replenish our physical and psychological resources. The dangers of chronic stress were discussed in chapter 3 and we know that in certain situations such pressure may have a serious effect on our health. Certain kinds of stress are obviously worse than others, and in particular aggressive stress or high levels of hostility appear to be associated with a much higher incidence of coronary heart disease.'

Dr Redford Williams, Professor of Psychiatry at Duke University in North Carolina, has claimed that there is a specific component of the 'Type A' personality which predisposes to heart disease. This component is a sense of angry hostility towards others, a belief that most people will lie, or be mean to you, rather than be nice. This sort of anger and hostility is particularly harmful when it is supressed and directed inwardly, as it often is. Many people feel a sense of mistrust and hostility towards others, a feeling which in fact stems from a basic insecurity and a lack of self-esteem. Anger generated in this form must be sublimated in one way or another, but preferably in a way which is socially acceptable. After all, you may dislike and distrust your boss but trying to sublimate your feelings by running him down in your car is likely to bring other pressures to bear upon you!

Many individuals find meditation a useful way of relieving stress, and others have hobbies such as painting or fishing which help to relieve the tension. What we choose to do matters not so much as the fact that we *do* find something of interest which we can use as 'therapy'. Most people who engage in physical exercise on a regular basis will tell you that they experience a tremendous sense of well-being, and particularly that they find it an extremely effective way of controlling and sublimating tension, anger and other stresses and strains.

In particular, many who run, swim or cycle regularly say that exercise is a wonderful way of channelling suppressed aggression. This question of the damaging effect of inwardly directed hostility towards others has been confirmed in a number of studies. In the late 1950s more than 1,800 men aged between 40 and 50 years employed by the Western Electric Company in the USA were evaluated with questionnaires that included certain questions designed to assess levels of hostility. Analysis of these data some 20 years later showed that of those who would be rated as low on the hostility scale only 18 per cent had died. The death rate among those on the high end of the scale was 26–30 per cent. According to Dr Williams, this is a measure of the effect of hostility on survival. He also evaluated a group of 255 medical students for levels of hostility, based on question-naires applied some 25 years previously. By the time they had reached 45–50 years of age, only two to three per cent of the low hostility group had shown evidence of coronary disease, compared with nine to twelve per cent of the high hostility group. This difference, which is greater than that found in the Western Electric study, does seem to suggest that high levels of anger and hostility could be an important factor in causing premature death from heart disease. Whether it is hostility, some other component of a particular form of behaviour or, more probably, a combination of a large number of factors, chronic stress needs to be sublimated in one form or another.

If we accept that we cannot always change our environment, our working conditions or our working colleagues, then we realize that the only factor we can effectively alter is our own reaction to our surround-ings. One effective way of managing stress and its consequences is to spend time exercising.

Although it has been known for many years that people who are physically fit and healthy experience an enhanced sense of well-being – a quality of life which it is extremely difficult to define – it has tended to be dismissed by the sceptics as yet another expression of a rather strange personality type commonly found among people who exercise. However, the discovery, in 1974, of a group of opioid peptides,* subsequently referred to as the 'endorphins', had major implications upon our under-standing of the psychological effects of exercise.

Perhaps there really was a basis for this feeling of wellness, that could be quantified in terms of changes in brain biochemistry? Perhaps the sense of elation and increased perception that some claim to experience during exercise could be accounted for in terms of increased levels of brain endorphins?

The endorphins themselves have a chemical structure which is similar to morphine, and as they are produced by the body itself, speculation soon grew that this group of substances was the 'natural' pain-killer or analgesic of the body.

The precise physiological role of the endorphins remains unclear, and possible associations with certain alterations in conscious level etc. are purely speculative at this stage. In 1980, however, Pargman and Baker developed the hypothesis that the endorphins are involved in producing

* These are proteins which have a similar chemical structure to opium or morphine.

the psychological adaptation called the 'runner's high', which is experienced by certain long-distance runners. This 'high', or feeling of elation, is variously described as a euphoric sensation or an 'altered state of consciousness'. This postulated role for endorphins was based upon evidence that they can produce an altered state of consciousness in which there is a reduction in responsiveness to external stimuli.

This is actually supported by the statements of many who are involved in regular endurance exercise who claim that they become almost completely unaware of the environment in which they are exercising. Somehow, the constant sense of movement and the exertion of running or cycling etc. produce a dissociation from the environment. Marathon runners in the final stages of a race often say that they have no recollection of the last six miles or so, despite the fact that in any physiological or medical sense they would normally be feeling extreme discomfort. It is possible that this ability to become detached from normal sensations of pain and discomfort is a function of chemical changes mediated in the brain by certain transmitters that block the normal pain sensation. The endorphins, or other chemicals, may also bring about an altered state of consciousness in which one's perception of the environment could be changed. Perhaps this is the 'runner's high'. Certainly Mandell (1979) has postulated that endorphins bring about a release of a substance called serotonin, which acts upon the limbic system in the brain producing alterations in consciousness.

It is likely that the endorphins act in concert with other complex chemical transmitters, such as catecholamines (adrenalin and noradrenalin), to produce changes in perception and consciousness. There is also some evidence that endorphins may effect other hormones during exercise. Endorphins have been shown to produce an increase in growth hormone and prolactin, and it is becoming clear that the actions of endorphins, and particularly their interactions with other hormones, are exceedingly complex.

It is clear, however, that levels of endorphin would have to increase during exercise if the interactions and responses we have mentioned are to be mediated. Appenzeller and others (1980) have demonstrated an increase in beta-endorphin as a result of long-distance running, suggesting that the speculation may have some basis in fact.

Other chemical transmitters are likely to be discovered as a result of future research, and we have yet to clarify the interactions between many already recognized transmitters and hormones such as adrenalin, noradrenalin, serotonin and dopamine, all of which have important effects on the brain.

It is interesting to consider whether the production of endorphins and related substances as a result of exercise may be related to the addictive quality of exercise, which we have mentioned previously. Exercise certainly has a compulsive quality about it for many people and some individuals display a sense of compulsion which can only be adequately described as an addiction. We certainly know that people become addicted to morphine and its derivatives, such as diamorphine (heroin). It is conceivable, therefore, that certain individuals may become addicted to their own endorphins. Furthermore, some individuals who have been forced to discontinue regular exercise experience symptoms such as irritability, insomnia and depression. Are these symptoms produced by withdrawal from endorphins or other substances produced within the body as a result of exercise? This is an interesting speculation.

It seems quite possible, therefore, that the benefits of exercise in reducing stress and bringing about a whole range of psychological benefits may have a basis in biochemical changes within the brain substance. Not everyone, however, who engages in exercise experiences the 'runner's high' or a similar state. Many have never experienced such benefits, even after many years of endurance training. In addition, some workers reject the hypothesis that endorphins have anything to do with such feelings. McMurray from North Carolina rejects the endorphin hypothesis, and believes that the 'runner's high' may be related to adrenalin or changes in blood gases as a result of overbreathing during exercise. He claims that many runners tend to hyperventilate (overbreathe), sometimes after a relatively short period of a few minutes, and this may produce a mild euphoric state. Other studies on runners have suggested that endurance and exercise intensity have no direct effect upon endorphin levels within the body.

Finally, other workers have suggested quite different explanations for the psychological changes resulting from exercise. Kostrubala has suggested that running or similar endurance exercises may bring about a relative change in the dominance of the brain hemispheres. The left side of the brain (the left cortex) is associated with logical and analytical thought, whereas the right cortex is more associated with abstract and creative thinking. It may be that as a result of endurance exercise, the right cortex assumes a temporary dominance, bringing about certain changes in perception.

Whatever the underlying mechanism, it is evident that physical activity can make substantial contributions to stress control and an enhanced sense of well-being. Those who work in this field cannot fail to be impressed by the testimony of individuals from all walks of life who describe the powerful psychological benefits of exercise. Some have even described the effects as a quasi-religious or mystical experience, although it must be said that few experience such profound revelations. Most people who exercise are aware that it offers an important means of sublimating tension and stress which are the hallmarks of an increasingly pressurized society. Quite simply, exercise makes you feel good. The fact that we cannot explain the mechanisms involved in such psychological changes should not detract from the powerful potential effects of regular exercise in bringing about such changes. After all, one does not need to be a highly trained motor mechanic to enjoy driving, and you do not need to have a rational, scientifically based explanation of the biochemical changes occurring in the cerebral cortex and other areas of the brain to feel a sense of enjoyment and improved quality of life from exercise.

Conclusions

We can summarize this discussion by listing the possible mechanisms by which exercise provides protection against coronary heart disease as including improved cardiovascular efficiency, direct effects on the coronary arteries themselves, reduction in blood pressure, beneficial alterations in blood lipids (fats), reduced blood sugar levels and better 'stress' control. This impressive list of benefits is outlined in figure 5.1. In chapter 7 we shall be discussing the frequency, duration and intensity of exercise required to bring about such changes, and also examining the forms of exercise that would seem appropriate.

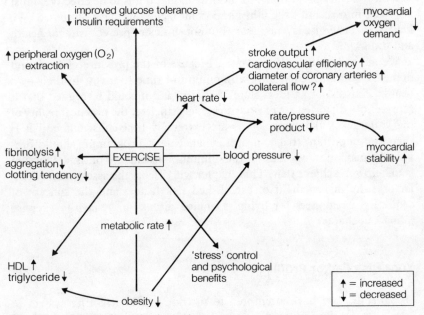

Figure 5.1   Effects of sustained exercise.

6

Acquiring a 'Readiness for Living'

In this chapter we shall be giving you practical advice about how you can assess the risks to your health and incorporate a simple and yet comprehensive health maintenance programme into your own lifestyle. Throughout this book so far we have emphasized the key role which regular exercise has to play in disease prevention and health maintenance. This is not because exercise is the only factor nor necessarily the most important one. It has been emphasized because hitherto, in the context of its relationship to disease, exercise has been either neglected or misunderstood.

However, any programme for healthy living, if it is to be effective, must also take into account the other important factors we have discussed. We believe that exercise is a necessary but not sufficient prerequisite for health and fitness.

We are aware that many people, because of the pressure of work and domestic commitments, have a minimum of time to invest in their own health. This is not an ideal state of affairs, and it could be argued that it represents a distorted set of priorities. Nevertheless, the practical reality of the situation is that most of us are extremely time-conscious and it is therefore important that a 'health enhancement' programme should provide the maximum rewards for the minimum investment of time. Our aim is to help you achieve that. This chapter will discuss the assessment of risk factors, the management of established risk factors and the concept of acquiring a readiness for living. Detailed discussion of *how* to exercise follows in chapter 7.

Your Risk Factor Profile

In figure 6.1 we have attempted to provide a points scoring system to assess six cardiovascular disease risk factors. The information you will

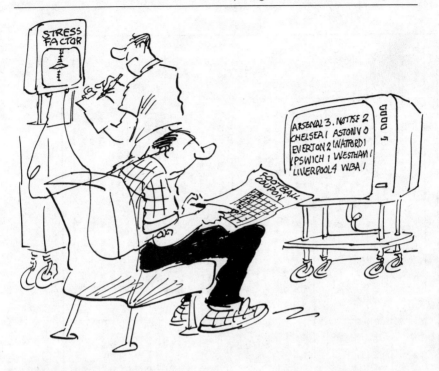

require to complete the assessment can be obtained by undertaking a two-stage screening procedure.

1st Stage – Self-screening

1 Cigarette smoking
2 Body weight
3 Physical activity
4 Stress and personality

These four factors should be considered and the appropriate scores entered. Cigarette smoking is straightforward. Simply estimate the number of cigarettes smoked daily and enter the appropriate score.

There are several methods of assessing your body weight. One of the most common methods is to look at the tables prepared by various insurance companies, notably the Metropolitan Life Assurance Company. These tables are based on studies of hundreds of thousands of insured men and women. There are a number of disadvantages to this approach, not the least of which is the fact that they require a method of classification into small, medium and large frame size.

Factor	Rating					Score
Cigarette smoking	None	Up to 9 daily	10–24 daily	25–34 daily	35 or more daily	
Score	0	1	2	3	4	
Blood Cholesterol	Less than 3.8 mmol/l (150 mg/100 ml)	3.8–4.3 mmol/l (150–169 mg/100 ml)	4.4–5.1 mmol/l (170–199 mg/100 ml)	5.2–5.6 mmol/l (200–219 mg/100 ml)	5.7 mmol/l or greater (220 mg/100 ml)	
Score	0	1	2	3	4	
Blood pressure (systolic)	Less than 110 mm of Hg	110–129 mm of Hg	130–139 mm of Hg	140–149 mm of Hg	150 mm of Hg or above	
Score	0	1	2	3	4	
Self-rating of stress/ personality tension	You are calm and serene about most things and rarely get upset or anxious. You have good relations in your job and with your family.	You are calmer than average. You may get a little upset when delayed but not unduly so. You have a fairly routine job with regular hours. You get upset with your family only occasionally.	Your emotional response and personality are balanced. You may feel tense or anxious two to three times a day. You rarely use tranquillizers or sedatives. You get upset and annoyed with your family when you have good reason to be.	You are usually rushed and are more aggressive than average. You are ambitious. You have a managerial or other demanding job. You get impatient when you feel things are moving too slowly. You have an above normal tendency to become emotionally upset and you may take the occasional tranquillizer or sedative.	You are extremely tense and very aggressive. You are very ambitious with a highly demanding job. You are very impatient in slow traffic etc. You are often very upset and annoyed, both at work and with your family. You may take sedatives or tranquillizers frequently.	
Score	0	1	2	3	4	
Body weight	Ideal weight	Up to 9 lbs (4 kg) overweight	10–19 lbs (4.5–8.5 kg) overweight	20–30 lbs (9–13.5 kg) overweight	More than 30 lbs (13.5 kg) overweight	
Score	0	1	2	3	4	
physical activity	Vigorous* exercise four or more times per week, for at least 20 minutes each	Vigorous exercise on three occasions each week for at least 20 minutes each.	Vigorous exercise on one or two occasions per week, for at least 20 minutes each.	Occasional exercise but nothing on a regular basis. Your leisure time is mainly sedentary.	You do essentially no exercise, do little walking and spend most of your working and leisure time, sitting.	
Score	0	1	2	3	4	

* Vigorous exercise should be regarded as forms of exercise which are regular and rhythmical, and involve major muscle groups.
Examples: Cycling, swimming, running, jogging, tennis etc. The activity should be continued for at least 20 minutes.
Brisk walking would qualify, provided it is brisk and maintained for at least 30 to 40 minutes.

Figure 6.1   Risk factor profile chart.

This is a modification of a scoring system prepared by John W. Farquhar and members of the Stanford Heart Disease Prevention Programme.

Table 6.1 Acceptable body weights according to height

Height without shoes (m)	Men			Women		
	Acceptable average	Acceptable range	Obese	Acceptable average	Acceptable range	Obese
1.45				46.0	42–53	64
1.48				46.5	42–54	65
1.50				47.0	43–55	66
1.52				48.5	44–57	68
1.54				49.5	44–58	70
1.56				50.4	45–58	70
1.58	55.8	51–64	77	51.3	46–59	71
1.60	57.6	52–65	78	52.6	48–61	73
1.62	58.6	53–66	79	54.0	49–62	74
1.64	59.6	54–67	80	55.4	50–64	77
1.66	60.6	55–69	83	56.8	51–65	78
1.68	61.7	56–71	85	58.1	52–66	79
1.70	63.5	58–73	88	60.0	53–67	80
1.72	65.0	59–74	89	61.3	55–69	83
1.74	66.5	60–75	90	62.6	56–70	84
1.76	68.0	62–77	92	64.0	58–72	86
1.78	69.4	64–79	95	65.3	59–74	89
1.80	71.0	65–80	96			
1.82	72.6	66–82	98			
1.84	74.2	67–84	101			
1.86	75.8	69–86	103			
1.88	77.6	71–88	106			
1.90	79.3	73–90	108			
1.92	81.0	75–93	112			

The heading *Weight without clothes (kg)* spans the Men and Women columns.

The report on obesity from the Royal College of Physicians published in 1983 sets out the reasons for considering a weight range for each height, sex and age group as appropriate for maintaining health. The weight ranges for adults are listed in table 6.1, which does not include any adjustment for frame size. In addition, these values do not include any adjustment for age, the implication being that adults should remain within the weight range throughout adult life. There is no good medical or physiological reason why any individual should weigh more at the age of 40 than at the age of 20. In fact, since body muscle mass diminishes with age, and since muscle is denser than fat, the body weight should actually decrease.

The weights are given in kilogrammes and the height is measured in metres. Table 6.2 shows the height in feet and inches and the weight in pounds.

Table 6.2   Acceptable body weights according to height

Height without shoes (ft in)	Weight without clothes (lb)					
	Men			Women		
	Acceptable average	Acceptable range	Obese	Acceptable average	Acceptable range	Obese
4′ 9″				101	92–117	141
4′ 10″				102	92–119	143
4′ 11″				103	95–121	145
5′ 0″				107	97–125	150
5′ 1″				109	97–128	154
5′ 1½ ″				111	99–128	154
5′ 2″	123	112–140	169	113	101–130	156
5′ 3″	127	114–143	172	116	106–134	161
5′ 4″	129	117–145	174	119	108–136	163
5′ 5″	131	119–147	176	122	110–141	169
5′ 5½ ″	133	121–152	183	125	112–143	172
5′ 6″	136	123–156	187	128	114–145	174
5′ 7″	140	128–161	194	132	117–147	176
5′ 8″	143	130–163	196	135	121–152	183
5′ 9″	146	132–165	198	138	123–154	185
5′ 9½ ″	150	136–169	202	141	128–158	189
5′ 10″	153	141–174	209	144	130–163	196
5′ 11″	156	143–176	211			
6′ 0″	160	145–180	216			
6′ ½ ″	163	147–185	222			
6′ 1″	167	152–189	227			
6′ 2″	171	156–194	233			
6′ 3″	174	161–198	237			
6′ 4″	178	165–205	246			

There is a fairly wide weight range for each height and this takes into account variations in frame size. The acceptable average weight is given in the left hand column. If your weight is above the upper figure in the acceptable range, then you should insert the appropriate number of points on your risk factor profile. For example, in the case of a male at 1.7 m, the acceptable weight range is 58–73 kg. If you are 6 kg over this limit, i.e. 79 kg, then you will enter a score of 2 on the risk factor profile chart. In the case of a woman at 1.62 m the acceptable weight range is 49–62 kg. If you actually weigh 72 kg you are 10 kg above the top of the acceptable range and you should therefore enter a score of 3 on the risk factor profile chart. In the table of acceptable weights you will see a series of figures in the right hand column headed 'Obese'. If your body weight is at this level or above then you would undoubtedly be classified as obese. For example, if you were a male at a height of 1.72 m and a weight of 89 kg, you would be classified as obese and you would enter a score of 4 into the risk factor profile chart.

You should bear in mind that the figures quoted are for an acceptable range of weights, and do not in any sense define a *desirable* weight. We shall be discussing the question of a desirable weight and weight reduction later in this chapter.

The scores for stress and physical activity patterns should then be completed. So far as the stress assessment is concerned, you may have some difficulty in finding one description that exactly matches your temperament and stress level. However, you should endeavour to rate yourself according to the description which you feel most closely approximates to the true one.

The section on physical activity should be quite easy to score, and there are notes to help you define more clearly what is meant by 'vigorous' exercise.

When you have completed your analysis of these four factors, you should then proceed to the second stage.

2nd Stage – General Practitioner Referral

At this stage you should visit your own family doctor for your blood pressure and blood cholesterol to be measured. The blood pressure is easily obtained by using an inflatable cuff and a sphygmomanometer. You should write down the value that your doctor provides for you, and enter the higher of the two values (systolic pressure). For example, if your blood pressure is 130/70, then the systolic blood pressure (130 mmHg) would require a score of 2 on the risk factor profile.

Measurement of your blood cholesterol should be fairly easy to accomplish since most general practitioners have access to regional laboratories. A blood sample is withdrawn after a suitable period of fasting (usually 12 hours) and the sample is then sent to the laboratory. A number of measurements will be made, including the level of the total cholesterol. You should then take this figure and enter the appropriate number of points on the chart. For example, if your blood cholesterol is 5.5 mmol/l (213 mg/100 ml) then you would enter a score of 3 on the risk factor profile chart.

You may feel reluctant to bother your doctor with what you may perceive as an unimportant or even trivial matter. However, we would emphasize that these matters are neither unimportant nor trivial and information on both these parameters may have a major bearing upon your long-term health prospects. Most general practitioners will, in fact, be pleased to assist you, although clearly some will be more cooperative than others. Some may not be at all cooperative, and may even refuse to assist you. If this is the case, then you should seek help elsewhere. Measurements of blood cholesterol and blood pressure take only a very small amount of time and in by far the majority of cases there will be no good reason for your doctor to refuse.

You will now have completed all the relevant sections of the risk factor profile and will be able to add up your total score. There are a total of six factors in all, and so the maximum score possible is 24 and the minimum score 0. Before analysing the scores it is worthwhile considering one or two other points. First, you will see that the chart does not contain any information concerning your family history, i.e., hereditary factors. This is because while a strong family history of coronary heart disease is significant, its influence does vary from individual to individual. Genetic factors, together with age and sex, are not amenable to change. For example, if you are male, aged 55, and both your parents died prematurely from heart disease, none of these risk factors can be influenced by anything that you do. It is, of course, all the more important therefore that you take note of any other risk factors which you may have and try your best to change them. All the risk factors included in our chart are at least potentially amenable to change.

You may also note that no mention has been made of the other biochemical factors discussed elsewhere in this book and which may be significant. For example, the level of high density lipoprotein (HDL), or fibrinogen. The reason for omitting factors such as these is not that they are not important, but that precise measurements of these substances are not easily obtainable and the evidence regarding their potential influence on the development of coronary disease is still accumulating. Finally, we have also had to take into consideration the question of simplicity. Entering every known risk factor on to the chart and allotting a potential score would make it unnecessarily complicated. Moreover, the reader should bear in mind that the chart and the total score obtained from it are only a guide and not an absolute indicator of the likelihood of problems in the future.

Score Analysis

Range 21–24 points

If you are in this category then you are at a substantially increased risk of suffering premature heart disease or a stroke. Indeed the probability of doing so is four or five times the national average. Urgent action is required and you must do everything you can to improve your risk factor profile. Those risk factors on which you have the highest scores, i.e. 4 or 3 points, should be attended to first.

Range 17–20 points

In this category your risk of a heart attack or a stroke is about two or three times the national average. You need to take urgent action to reduce your risk as much as possible. Attention should once again be paid to those factors on which you have scored the highest number of points.

Range 13–16 points

This range probably includes most people in this country. That is not to say that it is an acceptable range; indeed the reason the incidence of cardiovascular disease is so high is that we have hitherto been too complacent about the standards of health and fitness in this country. A minimum of effort could result in people in this range being classified into a much lower risk zone.

Range 9–12 points

This is a readily achievable level that would result in a substantial reduction in the risk of premature heart disease or stroke. In this range the likelihood of suffering one of these complications is about half the national average. That is not to say one should be complacent if one appears to be classified in this zone. There is always room for improvement.

Range 5–8 points

In this category the risk of a heart attack or stroke is about one-quarter of the national average. Achieving this points score takes considerably more effort, but the results are well worth it.

Range 0–4 points

In this category the incidence of heart attack and strokes is extremely low; indeed it may be as little as only one-tenth or one-twelfth of the national average. It will obviously take a great deal more time and effort to achieve, and not everyone will be able to do so because certain factors, for example blood cholesterol and blood pressure, can only be influenced to a certain extent by changes in diet and lifestyle.

While these scores are only a guide to the probability of your developing cardiovascular disease, they are nevertheless extremely important. Clearly if you have a total score of 22 or 23 points you will need to take decisive action to reduce your points score as soon as possible. Even reclassifying yourself into the range below will substantially reduce the likelihood of your developing problems. Most individuals will be capable of reclassifying themselves in the range below their present one with only a moderate amount of effort.

Do not become obsessed with the idea of achieving a zero rating. Few people, probably for genetic reasons, are capable of achieving such a low rating. Most of us, however, can achieve the range 9–12 points, and if all the members of our population were in this range there would be a major reduction in premature cardiovascular death and disability.

Finally we must stress that those individuals who find themselves in the highest points range and who therefore have a high risk of cardiovascular disease would almost certainly benefit from taking an exercise stress test prior to embarking upon a programme of physical activity. We recognize that the facilities available for this procedure are limited at the present time. Nevertheless if the opportunity is available, and you are able to undertake this procedure under expert cardiological supervision, then you should certainly take advantage of it.

Changing the Risk Factors

Now that you have carried out your initial risk assessment, we can set about giving you specific advice as to how to manipulate the individual risk factors.

Cigarette Smoking

The advice here is simple and straightforward. You should stop smoking immediately. Now you may argue that this is easier said than done and we fully appreciate the enormous difficulties that many individuals have in giving up this habit. However, we must state once again that without question it constitutes a major threat to your long-term health prospects.

Some of our patients have found help from acupuncture and hypnosis and some have also derived benefit from using nicotine substitutes such as nicotine-flavoured chewing gum. No doubt such methods have their place, but in our experience there are two absolute prerequisites for success if you wish to stop smoking. First you must make up your mind that you actually *do* want to stop. If you have not made up your mind about it, then you are unlikely to succeed. Secondly, you must have the determination and the willpower to implement your desire to stop smoking. Most of us have these qualities if we are prepared to look for them.

Pick a date and a time, think of yourself from that point on as a non-smoker, and make up your mind absolutely and completely that you will never touch a cigarette again as long as you live. Picture yourself refusing cigarettes when offered them. Picture yourself in enjoyable social surroundings without the cigarette in your hand. It is not an easy process but it can be achieved. Remember that the benefit to your health begins the moment you stop.

In our own practice we often encourage people to become involved in programmes of physical activity, weight reduction etc. and not to think too consciously about their cigarette consumption. Indeed, we often tell people not to consider this risk factor at all until after they have been involved in some regular physical activity and made the necessary dietary modifications. Often, after a period of say six weeks to two months, these individuals give up cigarette smoking quite easily. Having acquired a much better self-perception through improved fitness and reduced weight, they are often more able to see how inappropriate cigarette smoking is and what a harmful effect it will have upon their long-term health prospects. If an individual is running three or four times a week for 30 minutes, then at least during those periods he is not smoking. In addition, when he returns from his run, takes a shower and then sits down to eat a meal, he is much more likely to be conscious of how absurd it is to make the effort to go running and then come back and ruin the benefit by smoking a cigarette. Becoming involved in an exercise programme and changing one's diet is therefore often a useful and effective prelude to giving up cigarette smoking completely.

If, in the end, you are unable to give up cigarettes entirely, then there are still a number of things you can do in order to reduce your risk.

1 Smoke a low tar, low nicotine cigarette. Information about this is carried on every packet of cigarettes.
2 Try to smoke less of each cigarette and leave a longer stub. You should also make every effort gradually to reduce the amount you inhale in terms of both its frequency and its depth.
3 Switch to smoking a cigar or pipe and make every effort not to inhale the smoke.
4 Finally, try to set out some specific non-smoking times and venues. For example, do not smoke at home and do not smoke in the presence of your children. Do not offer anyone else a cigarette and if you must smoke then do it in the privacy of your own surroundings where you are unlikely to harm anyone else. The moment you walk into a crowded room with a cigarette in your mouth you become a health hazard. If this makes you feel uncomfortable and a social outcast, then so be it.

Blood Pressure

We have discussed blood pressure in detail elsewhere in this book. It is important to understand that there is no such thing as a 'normal' blood

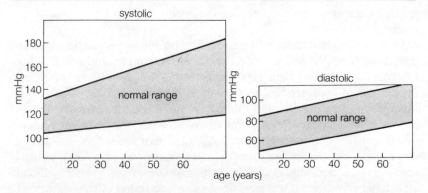

Figure 6.2   Systolic and diastolic blood pressure related to age.

pressure and it can be seen from figure 6.2 that blood pressure increases with age. This applies to both sexes. If your doctor tells you your blood pressure is elevated, there are a number of specific measures you can take to help improve the situation. If the level of your blood pressure is already such that there is evidence of a structural change in your heart and damage to other organs, then clearly treatment will need to be instituted immediately. In most cases this will be drug therapy and it may involve taking combinations of tablets.

In the majority of cases the blood pressure will not require immediate treatment. While in strict terms there is no such thing as a 'normal' blood pressure, there is an agreed cut-off point above which we regard a blood pressure as being significantly elevated. This level is a reading of 140/90 or above: clearly the higher the figures, the more significant the reading. If your blood pressure is found to be above this value, then there are several things you may do to improve the position, making drug therapy unnecessary.

Weight reduction

The association between overweight and high blood pressure has been demonstrated in scores of studies. Amery and his colleagues reviewed six studies in patients with high blood pressure and concluded that a decrease in body weight of 1 kilogramme correlated with a decrease in blood pressure of 3 mmHg systolic and 2 mmHg diastolic with weight losses up to 10 kg. Data from the Chicago Coronary Prevention Evaluation Programme by Stamler and his colleagues showed a clear correlation between weight reduction and blood pressure reduction over a five-year period. This study suggested that regular exercise might aid the lowering of blood pressure by reducing obesity, but also that it might have a direct effect upon lowering blood pressure itself.

Salt restriction

There is good evidence, which is discussed elsewhere (see chapter 3) that certain individuals are 'salt-sensitive'. The reasons for this are not absolutely clear, but it is apparent that many people will experience a substantial reduction in their resting blood pressure after a period of salt restriction. Salt intake is to a large extent habitual, and even though many of us can do without salt at the table, there is still a mistaken notion that the addition of salt to ordinary cooking is an essential prerequisite to making food tasty and wholesome. This is nonsense. A period of cooking without salt will prove this quite clearly once you have managed to get over your initial period of salt craving. We believe the evidence for a general reduction in salt intake is compelling and certainly if your blood pressure is above normal you should make every effort to reduce your salt intake as soon as possible. You also need to look for occult sources of salt, and you should get into the habit of reading food labels to assess the salt content of items before you buy them.

Regular exercise

As intimated above, there is evidence that regular exercise in itself will have a direct effect on lowering blood pressure. This is in addition to the indirect effect it has in reducing obesity.

In summary, therefore, weight reduction and salt restriction accompanied by a regular, moderate exercise programme may well be sufficient to bring about a substantial fall in your blood pressure to within more acceptable limits. If this is not the case, and if after implementing these suggestions your blood pressure is still found to be significantly elevated, then you should without doubt be treated with the appropriate form of drug therapy. Managing blood pressure without drugs is infinitely preferable to taking drugs for years on end, and unless there is already evidence of damage to the heart and other organs, then most patients will be safe in first undertaking a trial of non-pharmacological management. If your blood pressure is quite significantly elevated, then your doctor may decide to put you on drug treatment for the time being in order to give you a measure of protection while the other measures of salt restriction, weight loss etc., are implemented. When you have lost the required amount of weight and reduced your salt intake, it may then be possible to reduce or even discontinue drug therapy to see whether your blood pressure is now adequately controlled. If it is, then you will not need to recommence your drug therapy. If it is not, then you will need to restart your medication, and probably on a long-term basis.

If you do find that you have to take tablets for your blood pressure you should not find this alarming. It is important that you take the medication regularly and in doing so you will substantially reduce your risk of future complications. Of course, you should still be vigilant about your salt intake and weight loss and there is no reason why you should not exercise moderately and continue to have an interest in your diet. Finally, it is absolutely imperative that you continue to have your blood pressure checked at regular intervals to ensure that it is adequately controlled. In most cases checks every six months will be adequate and your therapy can be adjusted as necessary.

High Blood Cholesterol (Hyperlipidaemia)

There are several types of blood lipid (fat) abnormalities and there seems little doubt that high blood cholesterol concentrations, whether in a population or in an individual, denote an increased risk of coronary heart disease. This is now beyond argument, although the converse of the hypothesis, i.e. that reducing blood cholesterol would necessarily be accompanied by a reduction in coronary heart disease, has been difficult to demonstrate. However, evidence from the American Lipid Research Clinics Program, published in 1984, demonstrated conclusively that reduction of serum cholesterol does produce a substantial reduction in the risk of coronary heart disease. It was estimated that reduction in total cholesterol of 25 per cent was accompanied by a 50 per cent reduction in coronary heart disease. These findings are of major importance and emphasize the need to reduce blood cholesterol concentrations in the population as a whole.

The question of blood lipid abnormalities and the relationship between cholesterol and high density lipoprotein (HDL) was discussed in chapter 3 (see also appendix 1). Obviously, the lower the blood cholesterol level and the higher the level of HDL, the better. If your blood cholesterol is substantially elevated, then you will need to take specific measures to reduce this to within more acceptable limits.

Again the question of 'normality' is difficult to assess. This is because blood levels of cholesterol exhibit a bell-shaped distribution within the population, without clear separation between abnormal and normal values. In other words, there is a broad range of cholesterol concentrations within an apparently healthy population. Since blood cholesterol concentrations are influenced by diet and other environmental factors, standards are established for each population under consideration. What is usually done therefore, is to set arbitrary statistical limits of normal concentrations based on the examination of large numbers of apparently healthy subjects of different ages. The cut-off limit that is usually used is the upper five to ten per cent found in apparently healthy individuals, and the quoted 'normal' range is usually about 3.4–7.5 mmol/l. However, a substantial amount of epidemiological evidence suggests that blood cholesterol concentrations that are 'normal' in a statistical sense, are not necessarily healthy. We cannot regard a population that is at present being decimated by coronary heart disease as a 'normal' population. Accordingly, many workers have suggested that the levels we regard as normal or acceptable are in fact much too high. There is evidence to support this notion in the Framingham study, where coronary heart disease was found to be quite rare among those whose total cholesterol concentration was below 3.86 mmol/l (150 mg%).

Normal values vary between laboratories but in this country, as mentioned above, they are usually stated as being between 3.4 and 7.5 mmol/l (132–290 mg%). We believe that the upper value for this figure, i.e. 7.5 mmol/l, is much too high. We recommend that all individuals with a blood cholesterol of greater than 6.2 mmol/l (240 mg%) should take specific measures to reduce their cholesterol and total saturated fat intake. In addition, any individual below the age of 20 whose blood cholesterol level exceeds 5.2 mmol/l (200 mg%) should take specific dietary measures to reduce it. In simple terms, the lower your blood cholesterol the better.

There is a definite correlation between the amount of fat in your diet and the level of your blood cholesterol. This has been well documented in several studies. There is also good evidence that making the necessary dietary modifications, can result in a substantial reduction (15–25 per cent) in your cholesterol level. Only in a minority of cases where the blood cholesterol remains high despite dietary measures, does drug therapy become necessary.

If your blood cholesterol is significantly elevated, then you should make every effort to modify your diet accordingly. You should reduce your intake of saturated fats by controlling your animal fat consumption, and you should also specifically avoid those foods which are known to be high in cholesterol. The cholesterol-lowering diet on p. 112 will provide you with some useful guidelines.

When you have been on this cholesterol-lowering diet for a month or so you should return to your doctor to have your blood cholesterol estimated once again. Hopefully there will be a substantial drop in the cholesterol level, but if there is not, you should remain on the diet for a further period of time, after which your blood lipids can once again be estimated. In most cases a satisfactory reduction in blood cholesterol can be achieved and no further treatment, apart from the low fat diet, will be required. In a small proportion of cases, however, diet alone may not be sufficient, and therefore the question of drug treatment for the elevated cholesterol may need to be considered. This is a specialized area which we need not discuss in detail here. However, since we know that all drugs have potential side

Cholesterol-Lowering Diet

The fats in food contain substances called fatty acids. These are of two types:

a) **Saturated** – these are contained in fats of animal origin, which are usually solid at room temperature, e.g. butter, lard and cream.

b) **Polyunsaturated** – these are contained in fats of vegetable origin, which are usually liquid at room temperature, e.g. corn oil.

It is the **saturated** fats which are strongly associated with coronary heart disease. **Polyunsaturated** fats, primarily of vegetable origin, are *not* associated with coronary heart disease and may even have a protective role.

Foods which have large amounts of saturated fat (principally animal in origin) tend also to have large amounts of cholesterol. Thus by generally reducing your intake of saturated fat, you will at the same time reduce your cholesterol intake. (NB: Cholesterol is found *only* in animal products.)

Avoid the following foods	Foods allowed
1 Whole milk, cream, cheese, ice cream, egg yolk,* butter, lard, dripping, suet, evaporated or condensed milk	1 Skimmed milk, low fat cottage cheese, low fat yoghurt, egg white, Flora or other suitable margarines,† vegetable oils, especially corn oil, sunflower oil, safflower oil, olive oil and sesame oil
2 Fatty meats, e.g. pork, duck, goose, sausages, luncheon meats, corned beef, bacon, salami, meat pies, pork pies, mutton (these foods are high in saturated fat and cholesterol)	2 Lean meat and poultry (remove skin from poultry)
3 Liver, shellfish, brains, sweetbread, fish roe, tripe, kidney (these foods are high in cholesterol)	3 Fish
4 Foods which contain egg yolk, e.g. rich cakes and pastries, mayonnaise.	4 Homemade cakes or pastries using Flora or corn oil and egg white instead of egg yolk and butter
5 Malted milk drinks, such as Ovaltine, Horlicks, etc.	5 Breakfast cereals, milk puddings (skimmed milk), cereals, spaghetti, rice, sago
6 Chocolate and sweets containing butter or milk, e.g. toffee, fudge and butterscotch, mincemeat and lemon curd	6 Mineral water and fruit juices
7 Tinned and packet soups, tinned meat	7 All fresh vegetables and fruit except avocado pear and olives
	8 Wholemeal bread, granary bread or crispbread

If you are overweight you should also cut down on the following foods: sugar, sweets and chocolate, preserves, biscuits, puddings, cakes, and fried foods.

* No more than 2–3 egg yolks per week
† e.g. Co-op Good Life, Marks & Spencer Superspread, St. Ivel Gold, Safeway Sunflower.

effects, the use of drugs should usually be considered only after at least six months of sustained effort to control the blood cholesterol by dietary means alone. Drug treatment should certainly be considered in the following groups of patients.

- Patients who already have heart disease.
- Patients who have strong family histories of heart disease.
- Patients with one or more of the other established risk factors besides high blood cholesterol, e.g. hypertension, diabetes or cigarette smoking.

Overweight and Obesity

Before discussing the problems associated with overweight and obesity, a word of clarification is required. The terms 'overweight' and 'obese' are not synonymous. Being overweight means that your body weight is above the acceptable weight range for your height and sex. When the degree of overweight becomes excessive, the term obese is used. For example, consider the acceptable weight ranges provided in tables 6.1 and 6.2. If you are a male at a height of 1.7 m and a weight of 65 kg, your weight lies within the acceptable range and you are neither overweight nor obese. If, however, you weigh 80 kg, you are above the acceptable average and are classified as overweight. But if you are 88 kg or greater, you will be classified as obese.

Such a classification has its uses, but from a practical point of view the differences are purely semantic. The fact is that overweight is nothing other than a milder degree of obesity. The terms overweight and obesity imply an excess of body fat: the difference between the two is simply a question of degree.

If we accept the terms for the present, however, we know that recent surveys suggest that a very substantial proportion of the adult population in this country weighs in excess of the acceptable ranges, i.e. is overweight. The prevalence of overweight increases from 15 per cent in the 16–19 year age group, to 54 per cent in men and 50 per cent in women in the 60–65 year age group. When we consider all adults, almost 40 per cent of men and 32 per cent of women are classified as overweight, with 6 per cent of men and 8 per cent of women being sufficiently overweight to be classified as obese.

Evidence from the Framingham study in the USA suggests that obesity is an independent risk factor for coronary heart disease. A report by the Royal College of Physicians suggests that even mild degrees of overweight are significant. Risks associated with excess weight are not confined to those who are substantially obese, because there is a progressive increase in morbidity and mortality which is apparent with even small increases in weight above the upper limits of the acceptable range. It follows that we need not only be concerned about those who will be classified as obese, but also those who will classified as only mildly overweight.

Overweight or obesity is associated with coronary artery disease, high blood pressure, high blood fats, diabetes and gallbladder disease. It is therefore a major public health hazard. Neither is this a problem that is confined to adults: obesity or overweight is now a serious health problem among children and an overweight child is more likely to become an overweight adult.

Of course we are all aware of the problems of being too fat. At least two-thirds of the adult women in this country are trying to lose weight at any one time and probably as many as one-third of the male population. They provide a captive audience for the plethora of slimming magazines and books which cram the shelves of our newsagents and bookshops. Despite all the 'expert' advice, 95 per cent of those individuals who manage to lose weight will eventually put the weight back on.

In simple terms, obesity or overweight can be defined as a condition in which there is an execessive amount of body fat. Unfortunately the measurement of body fat is difficult and the term 'excessive' is not amenable to precise definition. This makes for difficulties in applying general tables of 'ideal' weights to large populations. When considering the usual tables of weight according to body frame size etc., such as the Metropolitan Life Insurance weight tables, the reader should understand that these weights simply reflect the statistical probability of excess morbidity and mortality associated with weights in excess of those quoted. It would be perfectly possible to be within the acceptable weight range in these and other tables and yet still have a considerable excess of body fat. The figures in our tables (tables 6.1, 6.2) suggest an acceptable *weight range*, but it is possible to be within the acceptable weight range and still have an excess of body fat. The confusion has come about because of the failure to recognize that what is important is not how much one actually *weighs*, but rather what proportion of the body weight is lean body weight and what proportion is fat. For example, it would perfectly possible for your body weight to be within the acceptable weight range as quoted in the standard tables, and yet for that weight to be made up of 30 or 35 per cent fat, which is certainly excessive. What we need therefore is a method of assessing body fat on an individual basis.

There are several methods of estimating individual body fat percentage. The measurement of skin fold thickness is simple and quick and has the great advantage of providing a more direct estimate of body fat. The method involves the use of skin fold callipers to measure the thickness of subcutaneous fat at different sites. Those most often chosen are the fold of fat just below the shoulder blade, the back of the upper arm, the front of the upper arm, and the front of the abdomen. This is not a highly accurate method, but it does give at least a reasonable guide to the body fat percentage.

Laboratory methods for the measurement of body fat are complex and involved. Measurements of body density, total body water and of the total body potassium, are expensive and time-consuming, and could hardly be applied on a mass basis. Nevertheless, the importance of some individual assessment of body fat cannot be overestimated.

Given the problems we have discussed above, we would recommend that you first establish whether you body weight is within the acceptable ranges, as illustrated in the tables. If you are above the acceptable range for your height and sex, i.e. if you are overweight or obese, then you will obviously have to lose some weight. However, even if your weight is within the quoted acceptable range, you should still obtain some more precise information about the amount of body fat by applying some simple tests. We recommend that all individuals, irrespective of whether they are within the acceptable weight range or are classified as overweight or obese, should apply the following simple test.

Waist to hip ratio

Several studies have shown that a high waist to hip ratio is significantly associated with coronary artery disease, stroke and other causes of premature death. Men characteristically carry their excess fat on their bellies, whilst women tend to deposit the fat on the thighs and the hips. The excess risk appears to be in the male type of fat distribution. This means that it is not merely how much fat men and women are carrying that determines the risks relating to obesity, but where the fat tissue is deposited. It seems that those with 'abdominal' obesity are more at risk than those who have their fat tissue deposited peripherally on the thighs and hips. In other words, a pot belly is bad news, irrespective of whether you are male or female.

To calculate your waist to hip ratio simply measure your waist in a relaxed state and divide this measurement by your hip measurement. For example, if you are female with a waist measurement of 24 and a hip measurement of 36 your waist–hip ratio is 0.6. This is well within the acceptable range. On the other hand, if you are a male with a waist measurement of 42 inches and a hip measurement of 38 inches, then the waist–hip ratio is 1.1, which is outside the acceptable range. Ratios of 1.0 for men and 0.8 for women are the highest healthy ratios. If your waist–hip ratio is above this, then you clearly need to lose some weight.

Pinch test

At least half of the total body fat is found directly beneath the skin. The amount of this fat can be roughly assessed at several sites. Those most often chosen are the back of the upper arm, roughly half way between the shoulder and the elbow, around the waist and on the back, just below the shoulder blade. These layers should not be more than one-half to one inch thick. If on any of these sites you are able to grasp a skin fold which is more than one inch thick, then you are carrying an excess of body fat and should aim to lose some weight. This simple principle applies to both men and women.

Chest–waist difference

Unless you are significantly overweight, there will be a substantial difference between your expanded chest measurement and your waist measurement. Taking a deep breath you should measure your expanded chest size with the tape measure level and tight under the armpits. You should then measure your waist at navel height, with your stomach in a relaxed position (not sucked in or forced out). For women the expanded chest measurement should be approximately ten inches or more than the relaxed waist measurement. For men the expanded chest measurement should be at least five inches greater than the relaxed waist measurement.

When you have carried out these simple tests in conjunction with a rough assessment according to the acceptable weight ranges in table 6.1 or 6.2, you should have a rough idea of how much weight you require to lose. If you are classified as overweight, i.e. if your weight is above the upper limit of the acceptable range, then in the first instance you should seek to get your weight within the acceptable range. You can then use the above three measurements to obtain a more accurate assessment of your body composition. The vast majority of the adult population requires to lose at least a few pounds in weight, and so the following remarks will apply to this group as well as to those who are obese or overweight.

Losing weight

For most people losing weight is never an easy process. This is because the vast majority of people try to lose weight by dieting alone. All manner of diets exist, some of which are harmless and some of which are frankly dangerous. There is no need to embark upon any fad dietary regimes of any kind. Neither should you attempt 'crash dieting'. Many people decide that when they lose weight they are going to cut out virtually all sources of food and become extremely excited when after a few days or so they have managed to lose seven or eight pounds in weight. What they fail to realize is that what they are losing is not fat weight but simply glycogen and water. (Glycogen is the storage fuel in muscles, and by starving themselves these people simply deplete the muscles of glycogen and a similar volume of water.) When the period of crash dieting is over, the glycogen and water are replaced and the weight is regained. Weight loss of approximately two to three pounds a week is a much more sensible proposition, and this is likely to be a permanent feature.

In essence, the best way to lose weight is to combine a programme of regular, moderate exercise, with a low fat, high fibre diet. Trying to lose weight by using either one of these methods alone is never easy, but the combination is extremely effective. Most women fail to lose weight properly because they do not, as a rule, engage in regular exercise programmes. It has been known for many years that exercise raises the resting metabolic rate, i.e. the rate at which the body burns energy. Remember it is the combination of exercise and diet rather than either one individually which will produce the most effective results.

We have seen previously (chapter 3) that a number of distinguished bodies have recommended a reduction in the total fat consumption of the population as a whole. This is because of the clear association between diets that are high in saturated fats and coronary heart disease. A second reason for recommending a reduction in total fat intake is the problem of obesity. Fat contains more than twice the number of calories per unit than either carbohydrate or protein, and it follows therefore that if you wish to lose fat, you should reduce your total fat consumption. In general, therefore, we recommend a low fat, high fibre diet with some restriction of carbohydrate intake. The carbohydrate eaten should be complex carbohydrate, for example, pasta, rice, jacket potatoes, wholemeal bread. Those sources of carbohydrate which also contain large amounts of fat, for example, cakes, pastries etc., should be avoided. You will need to have some complex carbohydrate in order to fuel your exercise programme. Without this, you will become unduly fatigued while performing your exercise and will therefore lose the beneficial effect exercise has upon the metabolic rate.

There are many excellent books on the subject of low fat, high fibre cooking. Our brief, in this respect, is not to provide the detail but to set out the essential principles upon which a special diet should be based. We have set out overleaf a low fat diet which many of our patients have used with great success.

You should bear in mind that putting excess fat on is always easy, but removing it takes a great deal longer. You will need to be persistent and consistent in your efforts. Do not try to go for too dramatic a weight loss in

Low Fat Diet

Breakfast – same every day   1 slice dry wholemeal toast
Half a grapefruit
Tea with lemon or black coffee

Day One

Lunch   As many slices as you like of cold meat, e.g. turkey, lamb, chicken.
Tomatoes – as many as you want.

Dinner   Grilled fish with a combination salad, as many vegetables as you like.
1 slice wholemeal toast
1 grapefruit

Day Two

Lunch   Fruit salad, as much as you can eat

Dinner   Hamburger, lots of tomatoes, lettuce, olives, celery, Brussels sprouts, and cucumber

Day Three

Lunch   Tuna fish or salmon salad with lemon and vinegar dressing

Dinner   Two lamb chops, salad of celery, cucumber, tomatoes

Day Four

Lunch   Two boiled eggs, cottage cheese, 1 slice dry wholemeal toast

Dinner   Cold chicken, as many green vegetables as you can eat, e.g. spinach, cabbage

Day Five

Lunch   Assorted cheeses, 1 slice dry wholemeal toast

Dinner   Fish, combination salad, as many vegetables as you like
1 slice dry wholemeal toast

Day Six

Lunch   Fruit salad, as much as you can eat

Dinner   Cold chicken with combination salad
1 grapefruit

Day Seven

Lunch   Chicken with tomatoes, carrots, cabbage, broccoli or cauliflower
1 grapefruit

Dinner   Steak, tomatoes, celery, cucumber or boiled Brussells sprouts

Black coffee or tea with every meal

NB: Where red meat is included, it should be lean and you should remove any excess fat prior to cooking. Where poultry is included, the skin should be removed.

the first instance. Aim to achieve weight loss of approximately two to three pounds a week over a fairly long period. You will find eventually that your weight will tend to stabilize at a set level.

Finally, a word of caution. Do not become a slave to your dieting and do not become obsessional about achieving and maintaining the 'perfect' weight. There is an idea that healthy eating and healthy cooking must of necessity be rather boring, whereas nothing could be further from the truth. When you next have an opportunity, flick through the pages of some of the wholefood cookery books and you will be astonished at how exciting and attractive healthy eating can be. However, we all enjoy indulging ourselves occasionally, and so once in a while you should go to your favourite restaurant and pick what you most enjoy on the menu – even all the wrong things! Good food and wine, even rich food and wine, are very enjoyable and you should not feel guilty about an occasional self-indulgence.

After a suitable period of weight loss you should find that your body weight is within the acceptable range. The time it takes for you to achieve this will obviously depend upon how overweight you were in the first place. If you then find that your waist–hip ratio, the pinch test and the chest–waist difference are within the acceptable ranges, it is likely that your weight will be a close approximation to the 'ideal'.

Coping with Stress

Stress has come in for a great deal of bad publicity in recent years. We are bombarded by articles and television programmes devoted to the potentially lethal effects which stress may have upon us, and many people are left with the impression that stress of any kind is potentially harmful. As a result of all this publicity and increasing interest, stress management is now a new 'growth industry'. All this, however, is despite the fact that the term has never been adequately defined.

Hans Selye defined the stress phenomenon as the 'non-specific response of the body to any demand made upon it'. In other words, it is the body's natural and necessary reaction to any challenging situation. Definitions of this kind, however, are not very helpful. What constitutes a challenging situation to one individual may be almost totally disregarded by another. We also have to take into account that stress may be both psychological and physical, or even a combination of both. We also know that equivalent amounts of stress will have widely differing effects upon different individuals, and that differing *forms* of stress can have widely differing effects. Some people will crumble completely in situations that other individuals may not find in the least bit threatening.

There are two things we can say about the stress phenomenon at this point. First, what is common to all forms of adverse stress is that they contain an element of *threat* within them. It is the fear this implicit threat generates that leads to the stress. Our twentieth century environment contains a multiplicity of threats, most of which we are not actually conscious of most of the time. There is the threat of nuclear war – the greatest threat of all. There is the threat of illness as we get older. There is the threat of losing personal relationships and feeling lonely and isolated. There is the threat of losing our jobs and our financial security, or the threat of losing our own self-esteem because we have not achieved what we set out to achieve.

Secondly, we also know that too much stress can lead to physical illness and breakdown. There is a definite association between adverse life events and physical illnesses such as heart disease, hypertension, cancer, ulcers and bowel disorders. We do not know for certain how these stress responses become translated into physical illness, but the association between the two is clear. This is not to suggest that all people who are under stress would become physically ill; nor is the converse true, i.e., that all people who become ill have necessarily been exposed to stressful life events. As a generalization, however, it does appear to be the case that chronic anxiety and stress can lower your resistance to illness to the point where you become much more susceptible to physical and mental breakdown.

However, the idea that all stress is bad for you is a myth. Some of the most rewarding moments in our lives are moments of great stress. Indeed some stress is an absolute prerequisite to having a sense of fulfilment and excitement in life and learning how to manage stress can even be fun in itself. It is all a question of getting the balance right.

There are three main phases to the stress response, which Hans Selye termed the general adaptation syndrome (GAS). In the first phase there is an acute reaction by the body to the stressful stimulus, which results in the liberation of adrenalin and other stress hormones, which in turn increase the heart rate, the blood pressure and the respiration. These are normal physiological responses by which the body will respond to a potentially stressful or threatening stimulus.

In the second phase the acute reaction subsides and we enter a phase of resistance in which the body is held in a state of 'readiness' to respond. When properly managed, and when only sustained for certain periods, this state of readiness can be enormously productive. It is what gives us the impetus to achieve and to progress.

The third phase of the general adaptation syndrome, however, is potentially harmful. This occurs when the level of arousal or the state of readiness continues for too long, and a state of chronic exhaustion ensues. It is often compounded by the fact that many individuals apparently do not have the ability to recognize this stage in themselves and will continue in this mode until illness, exhaustion or other factors compel them to stop.

Individuals in this tertiary stage may exhibit certain forms of behaviour which may be readily apparent to those around them. They are often bad tempered, argumentative and irritable. They may not eat or sleep properly, and their sense of exhaustion is compounded by the fact that they may turn to tranquillizers or other forms of sedation in an effort to cope. They may also increase their alcohol consumption as the stress syndrome continues. There may be inappropriate responses to events which at other times would be regarded as trivial.

One of the key points in effective stress management therefore is to learn to recognize phase three symptoms and to take heed of comments that others around you may make which may suggest that you are being exposed to an unacceptable amount of stress for too long.

There are basically two ways of coping with stress. Either we alter the environment in which we live and work to reduce the amount of stress to which we are exposed, or else we change our reaction to that imposed stress. From a practical point of view it is not easy to alter environmental sources of stress and therefore the only possible control we have is in our own reaction to that imposed stress. If you cannot actually change it, you can at least learn to cope with it more effectively.

The following points will perhaps provide a useful framework in which you can begin to manage stress more effectively and turn it into something that is positive and even enjoyable.

1 Learn to recognize signs of exhaustion and stress in yourself. Listen carefully to what others around you, particularly family and friends, may say about your mood and your appearance. They may notice a change for the worse long before you do.

2 Learn to say 'No'. When you honestly cannot make a particular meeting or a deadline or become involved in yet another project, a clear simple 'No' is the best and the most sensible option.

3 Effective organization can be a powerful means of achieving control over your own life. If you are habitually late for work and sit in traffic jams biting your nails while your blood pressure rises because you know you are going to be late *again*, then you are not being organized. Leaving home 15 minutes earlier can make all the difference and this may mean that you should get up a little earlier. Perhaps you are not able to get up in the morning because you spend too much time late at night watching television, perhaps even programmes in which you are not even remotely interested. Is it really that difficult to turn off the television and go to bed half an hour earlier? So many of our activities are habitual and one has to

learn how to recognize habits of this kind and deal with them effectively.

4 Make sure you have a suitable leisure time interest or hobby, preferably one which you can share with other people. Be interested in something and you will be interesting. If you are interested only in your job and are incapable of talking about anything else, you will become a bore.

5 Try your best to set aside a regular exercise period of three or four occasions per week. Saying that you cannot manage it or you simply do not have time is really not good enough. The point is that you have to make it a priority and recognize that regular exercise and its benefits is not some form of chore which you have to perform because it is a good idea. Neither is it something you should do only when and if you have the time. You have to change your perception of the role of exercise in your life and make it a priority. The benefits are very substantial, both in terms of increased working efficiency and also in stress management. Most people can find three or four 20-minute periods during the week which they can devote to exercise. The claim that they cannot do so is nothing other than laziness and if they really *cannot* find three or four 20-minute sessions during a seven day week, then there is something radically wrong with the way in which they are living and organizing their lives.

6 Do try to share your problems and your anxieties with those around you. The old adage that a 'trouble shared is a trouble halved' is absolutely true. There are no points awarded to those who carry their burdens in splendid isolation. It is not martyrs we want, it is effective communication.

7 However busy and committed you are to your work or your other interests, do try to listen to the needs of those around you. It may mean that on occasions you have to compromise to accommodate others, and this is not always easy or even possible. Nevertheless, the fact that you have listened and more importantly *heard* what has been said to you is extremely important.

8 Remember that the corporation/company/organization etc. will continue to function without you. Do not ever delude yourself by believing that you are irreplaceable. No one is that important.

A final point, and perhaps the most important of all, do try to preserve a 'fail-safe' mechanism that will serve as your final protection. There must be an ultimate point at which you will simply switch the whole lot off and walk away from it. However irresponsible this may sound, and even though you may never actually reach that point, the fact that it exists and that you are prepared to use it can be a source of immense comfort! We all believe that our work is important, and we all like to believe that in some way we are indispensable, but this is not so and we do occasionally get matters out of perspective. Bertrand Russell wrote: 'One of the signs of impending madness is the belief that one's work is important. If I were a medical man I should prescribe a long holiday to anyone who believed that his work was important.' The secret lies in keeping a sense of balance and perspective both in terms of what we do and in the positions that we hold.

One eminent American cardiologist has said that there are two things and only two things to be learned about effective stress management. They are 'Number one – don't sweat over the small stuff. Number two – It's *all* small stuff!'

'Readiness for Living'

Before going on to discuss the practicalities of exercise in chapter 7, we want to discuss the concept of 'readiness for living'. We have decided to use this term rather than the more often used 'fitness' which has become abused and is largely misunderstood. Readiness for living is actually a much broader concept and does not carry with it the connotations of marathon running or other extreme forms of vigorous physical exercise.

A readiness for living is simply the ability to cope with the physical and mental demands of life. The term also gives us some idea of what fitness is for. Fitness is important in so far as it provides us with a readiness for living.

Readiness for living can be defined more precisely as the difference between the physical energy an individual has available to complete a task, and the fatigue imposed upon that individual at the time of performing that specific task. This is an extremely important concept to grasp and requires a little more explanation.

When an individual exercises he converts capital energy in the form of food to mechanical energy in the form of muscle and bone movement. The capital energy involved in muscle movement can be ascertained by measuring the heat liberated by the working muscles. This involves a time-consuming process using a calorimeter. Scientists have also demonstrated, however, that the measurement of oxygen consumed at rest, or during work, is equal to the heat produced as determined by the calorimeter. It follows that when we know the type of food consumed, that is carbohydrates, fat or protein, and the amount of oxygen used, we can express the energy needed to perform a task in the form of calories. In addition, by measuring the amount of oxygen used while performing a variety of work, we can then calculate the calorific value of each of these forms of work. In other words, we can quantify the amount of calories expended while digging the garden, cycling, swimming and performing a variety of other forms of physical activity.

During the past 20 years or so a number of scientists have obtained data for the calorific value of many industrial and leisure-time activities. This ability to quantify work accurately is extremely valuable when one is trying to match a person's ability to perform leisure activities with his own maximum energy expenditure. Our own laboratory equipment allows us to measure the amount of oxygen consumed by an individual, which, as we have seen, is directly related to the energy expenditure. The maximum oxygen consumption ($\dot{V}O_2$ max) measured therefore gives us an accurate estimate of an individual's ability to perform work.

We quantify maximum oxygen consumption in terms of units of energy, which we call METs. We define one MET of energy as the amount of energy used in the supine position in resting conditions. For example, sitting in a chair watching television will cost you approximately one MET of energy. Two METs would be twice the energy used at rest, and 17 METs, which is the energy required to play a hard game of squash, is 17 times the resting energy requirement. Using the $\dot{V}O_2$ max measurement we calculate MET capacity as follows:

$$\text{MET capacity} = [\dot{V}O_2 \text{ max (ml kg}^{-1} \text{ min}^{-1})/3.5\star$$

As an example, if the measured maximum oxygen consumption was 40.5 ml kg^{-1} min^{-1} then the MET capacity would be equal to 40.5/3.5 = 7.6 MET. If the $\dot{V}O_2$ max were 70 ml kg^{-1} min^{-1} then the MET capacity is equal to 70/3.5 = 20 MET.

Since we know the MET values of various forms of activity, it is possible for us, in the laboratory situation, to predict whether an individual would be capable of performing certain levels of physical activity in safety. The MET capacities for some of the most common activities are shown opposite.

This list is hardly exhaustive and is only meant to indicate the approximate MET values for certain activities. Clearly the potential MET range for each activity is enormous; for example, running at eight-minute mile pace is approximately 9–10 METs whereas running at five-minute mile pace is 20 METs. When classifying fitness in terms of METs, the average sedentary adult will have a MET capacity of approximately 9–10 ($\dot{V}O_2$ max 31.5 ml kg^{-1} min^{-1}). A three times a week jogger will have a MET capacity of approximately 15–17 ($\dot{V}O_2$ max 52.5–59.5 ml kg^{-1} min^{-1}). A

★ Since one MET is equal to 3.5 mls/kg/minute then the MET capacity is obtained by dividing the maximum oxygen consumption ($\dot{V}O_2$ max) by the figure 3.5.

Activity	METs
Rest (supine)	1
Dressing and undressing	2
Walking to 5 mph	3
Making beds	3
Cleaning windows	3
Level cycling (9.7 mph)	5
Chopping wood	6.5
Level walking (4 mph)	6.5
Badminton	5.8
Digging	7.5–9
Jogging	6–7
Level cycling (13 mph)	9
Level running (8 min/mile)	9
Level running (7 min/mile)	12
Squash	15–17

world class runner could have a MET capacity as high as 25 ($\dot{V}O_2$ max 85–90 ml kg^{-1} min^{-1}).

Returning now to our concept of 'readiness for living', we shall consider a sedentary individual with a MET capacity of 10 ($\dot{V}O_2$ max 35 ml kg^{-1} min^{-1}). If the work task undertaken by this individual requires the whole of his MET capacity, i.e., maximum effort, then the time for which this work could be continued would be assessed in seconds as opposed to hours. Obviously one can only work at maximum capacity for a very short period of time.

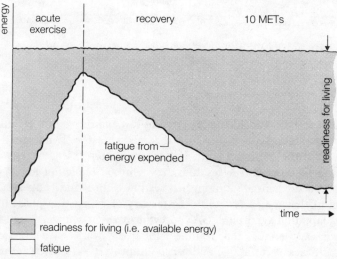

readiness for living (i.e. available energy)

fatigue

Figure 6.3   Energy expenditure and recovery from fatigue.

The fatigue imposed during this task would be maximal and immediately following this the readiness for living would be low. If the individual were asked to repeat this task he would fail and would require several hours to recover. During this recovery period the fatigue would decrease steadily while the physical capacity of 10 METs would remain constant, therefore the difference between physical capacity and the fatigue, i.e. the readiness for living, would increase. After a suitable period of recovery the task could be repeated. The situation is summarized in figure 6.3.

We have described an acute situation in which a heavy exercise load is applied in a very short period. However, a similar interaction between fitness (work capacity) and fatigue can be described for a 24-hour day. Fatigue increases throughout the day and the readiness for living (the available energy) steadily diminishes. Following a period of adequate rest and sleep the fatigue level diminishes and therefore the available energy, i.e. the readiness for living, will increase once again. This 24-hour cycle is illustrated in figure 6.4

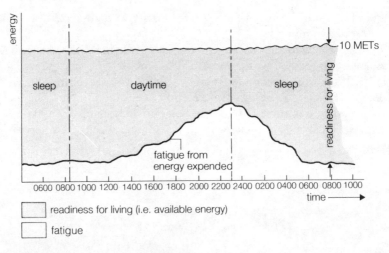

Figure 6.4 The 24–hour energy cycle.

It can be seen that an adequate period of rest and recovery is essential if the available energy, and therefore the readiness for living, are to be maintained at the optimum level. If, for any reason, this is not possible, fatigue can be cumulative, resulting in a chronic reduction in available energy and a substantially diminished readiness for living. This situation is typical of that which occurs in the tertiary or exhaustion phase of the general adaptation syndrome (GAS) previously discussed (see figure 6.5).

We can see therefore that readiness for living, varies as a function of individual fitness and fatigue and can be improved by an increase in the

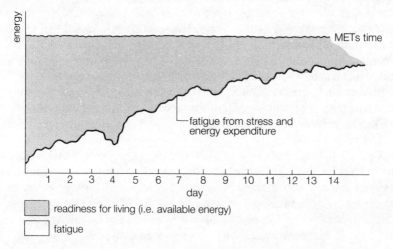

Figure 6.5 The effect of prolonged fatigue on readiness for living.

former, a decrease in the latter or a combination of both. In practice, it is not possible to reduce the fatigue imposed by everyday tasks since these are relatively constant. It follows that the most effective way to bring about an increase in readiness for living is to improve physical working capacity (fitness). This will automatically produce a relative decrease in the fatigue associated with everyday activities. A simple example will illustrate the point. Consider two individuals with MET capacities of 10 and 15 respectively, involved in a task requiring an energy capacity of 8 METs. We can see clearly that for the individual with 10 METs the task represents 80 per cent of his maximum energy and could therefore be maintained only for a short period. The relative fatigue is therefore

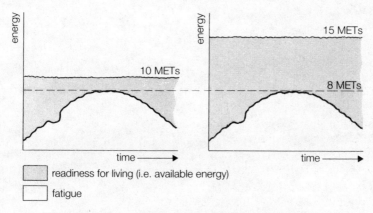

Figure 6.6 Effect of differing energy capacities (METs) on fatigue.

substantial. A significant recovery period will be required before the activity can be engaged in once again. However, for the individual with 15 METs this represents only 53 per cent of his total capacity and could potentially be continued for many hours. The *relative* fatigue is substantially less and therefore the readiness for living, or the available energy, is therefore much greater. It follows that while these two individuals are doing the same work, at the end of the week and during their leisure-time weekends, their readiness for living will be substantially different (figure 6.6).

We thus believe that the quality of life can be improved by increasing one's level of fitness or capacity to produce energy. The difference between fatigue and maximum energy is increased, giving life a new dimension. Enthusiasm and zest are a feature of the decrease in body fatigue facilitated by fitness. Even modest increases in energy capacity (METs) can make a very real difference to the relative fatigue imposed by everyday tasks.

7

How Should I Exercise?

Before discussing exactly how we should go about exercising, it is worth reminding ourselves, briefly, of what we have discussed. We have agreed that there is a need to improve our fitness in order to acquire a greater readiness for living. An increased MET capacity (energy capacity) will result in a relative reduction in fatigue levels for any given amount of work. Prior to commencing our exercise programme we will have completed our detailed questionnaire and will have already set about manipulating those other conventional coronary risk factors which we have identified.

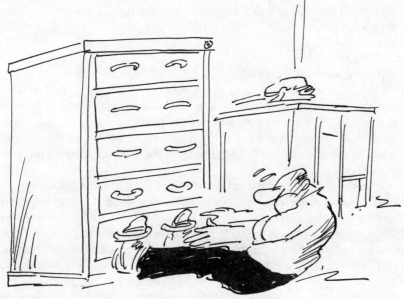

We are assuming that at this point you are yearning to add a new dimension to your life by improving your fitness. Having successfully completed a pre-exercise risk factor assessment you are now quivering on the doorstep correctly adorned in track suit and shoes and about to remove one of the great deficiency diseases from your life, i.e. lack of exercise. Bear in mind, however, that while we want you to exercise we do not want you suddenly to emerge from your world of gin and tonics, smoked-filled lounges, crème caramel and crêpe Suzette, tuck your 20 lb of excess adipose tissue into your running shorts and head for the hills. We do not want you to try to remove the inertia of 20 years' soft living in 30 minutes, because you may not be successful, and also you must remember that exercise has its dangers. These cannot be ignored, and we have discussed them in detail in chapter 9.

A few moments reflection will reveal that there is a simple, logical and structured way to proceed which will undoubtedly bring results. Let us consider the following four points:

- What type of exercise should I do?
- How often should I exercise?
- How hard should I exercise?
- For how long should I exercise?

We shall discuss each of these points separately and we will then be in a position to draw them together so that we can design an individual training programme.

What Type of Exercise?

We must make it absolutely clear at the outset that when we talk about fitness, i.e. the capacity for work, we are talking about increasing *cardiovascular* efficiency. It is the improvement in the efficiency of the heart and lungs which is paramount, since it is this which brings about an increased readiness for living.

Exercise is usually classified into dynamic, static and a combination of both. Dynamic exercise involves major muscle groups, is regular, rhythmical and brings about a substantial increase in heart rate and respiration. This is sometimes referred to as 'aerobic' exercise. Static exercise, on the other hand, involves individual muscle groups for relatively short periods and does not tend to produce an increase in heart rate or respiration in the way that dynamic exercise does. Weight training, for example, is a form of static exercise. In terms of developing cardiovascular fitness it is generally assumed that dynamic exercise is significantly superior to static exercise.

Indeed many people question the value of long-term static exercise and suggest that the high blood pressures induced could be dangerous. This would obviously be particularly relevant for those individuals who are already classified as hypertensive. However, static exercise is quite effective in increasing muscle strength and in some joint injuries it is the only way that muscle wasting can be prevented.

In terms of developing cardiorespiratory fitness, dynamic exercise involving large muscle groups is required for maximum effect. Examples of this form of exercise are running, jogging, cycling, swimming, rowing and brisk walking. However, the reader must remember that the heart is simply a pump working inside a closed system and it therefore has no ability to discriminate between various activities; therefore, if the above criteria for cardiovascular exercise are being met, the type of exercise is totally irrelevant. The most important thing is that you should choose an activity which you enjoy and which you are therefore likely to comply with. If you are to achieve a measure of success, it is vital that you should perform the exercise regularly throughout the week. If you do not basically enjoy the exercise then you are hardly likely to achieve this.

We would certainly suggest that any individual who is obese should commence his exercise programme with non-weight-bearing exercise such as swimming, cycling or the use of a rowing machine or stationary exercise bicycle. This will enable a substantial increase in cardiovascular fitness and will also help to promote weight loss, as we have mentioned earlier. This improvement in cardiovascular efficiency, coupled with weight loss, can be achieved with a minimum risk to joints and tendons since weight is being adequately supported by other means. When the body weight has been normalized, then jogging, running, skipping and many other weight-bearing activities can be added safely to the training schedule.

Many people who are not obese at the commencement of training would prefer the simplicity of donning a pair of running shoes and shorts and running along the pathways of a favourite beauty spot. The type or mode of exercise is not important, nor is one particular exercise intrinsically superior to another. However, differing forms of exercise may have particular advantages for certain temperaments and lifestyles and it is worth considering some of these in more detail so as to illustrate these points. Let us consider running/jogging, swimming and cycling, all examples of highly effective dynamic exercise.

Running/Jogging

There is no doubt that regular running/jogging is an excellent form of cardiovascular exercise. What exactly constitutes jogging as opposed to running is difficult to define, although it is usually taken that jogging is slower and less vigorous than running. Few people would argue that if you can cover a mile inside five minutes you are running as opposed to jogging. Conversely, if you take 10 or 12 minutes to cover the same distance, then one would regard that as jogging. It follows that at some point between a five- and ten-minute mile, jogging merges into running, but the point at which one transforms into the other cannot be defined, and quite frankly, the discussion is of no practical consequence. If one chooses to jog/run as a form of exercise, then it is the duration and the intensity which matters rather than the name you give to it.

A more important consideration is the question of what sort of footwear you should use. Nowadays, there is a bewildering choice of footwear available and the technology and expertise utilized in the design and manufacture of running shoes has been refined considerably during the past decade or so. The specific brand name you choose is entirely a personal choice. Most of the larger companies will have shoes to fit your requirements. However, you should, where possible, obtain expert guidance, which should be available at your local sports shop. The most important thing, obviously, is that the shoe should fit adequately. You should bear in mind that as the foot hits the ground a certain amount of distortion takes place and the foot in effect 'spreads' through the shoe. This means you will need shoes that are slightly larger than usual to give your foot the room in which to expand. This means there should be between one-quarter and three-quarters of an inch between the big toe and the end of the shoe. If one foot is larger than the other then you should choose a larger size, and do not forget to use the 'standing' rather than the 'sitting' size of the foot as the most accurate.

Wearing the correct footwear for running/jogging is absolutely crucial and this point cannot be emphasized enough. During a ten-mile run each shoe will land on the ground 10,000 times, and for an average person weighing 170 lb this will mean that a cumulative force of between 700 and 800 tons will be delivered through the shoe during that ten-mile run. This potentially places tremendous stresses upon the feet, ankles, knees, hips and spine and if you do not wear the correct type of footwear you will almost inevitably develop orthopaedic problems. Cushioning and stability are, without question, the key factors. Prevention is always better than cure. A wise investment at the outset may save you a great deal of trouble.

There are several clear advantages to choosing running/jogging as opposed to other forms of exercise. First, there is the question of convenience. You can basically run anywhere and at any time, provided that the surface is good enough and, if it is winter, the area is adequately lit. If your job involves a great deal of travelling, then nothing could be easier than simply to throw your running shoes into the back of the car or into your travelling case and take them with you. Although the running shoes may be fairly expensive, the overall investment in this form of exercise is actually extremely small. The average pair of running shoes may last you 12 months to two years, so spread over that sort of time the investment is not a large one. If you can afford it, then it is certainly worthwhile purchasing a good quality tracksuit which, if well cared for, should last for several years. So running is extremely effective, convenient and relatively inexpensive.

There are several disadvantages which we also need to mention. The most common complaint about jogging/running as a form of exercise is that many people find it extremely tedious. There is really no easy way around this. You either basically enjoy or are prepared to tolerate the exercise or you are not. If running is not for you then you should obviously seek some other form of exercise which you are more likely to comply with. The second point is that if you are substantially overweight, then running may precipitate problems with your Achilles' tendons, ankles, knees and hips. This is why we have stressed that if you are overweight a non-weight-bearing form of exercise would be more appropriate in the early stages until your weight has been reduced. Not only will this improve the cardiovascular state prior to the commencement of your running/jogging programme, but it will also significantly improve the strength and condition of the leg muscles, making orthopaedic injuries very much less likely. Again, we would emphasize that the correct choice of running shoes is extremely important in the prevention of such injuries.

One or two other natural hazards are worth mentioning. If you run along pavements look out for pot-holes and also for low level branches from trees and shrubs. If the area in which you run is not well lit in winter time then branches at head and particularly eye level can be potentially dangerous. If you live in the city then you will have to choose your running/jogging time with great care. Quite frankly, running in rush-hour traffic with all the fumes and grime is likely to do you more harm then good. The air is heavily laden with chemicals and carbon monoxide, and since the latter is at least a hundred times more soluble in blood than oxygen, the level of carbon monoxide in the bloodstream will rise proportionately. Added to this you have the risk of being seriously injured or killed on the roads, particularly as motorists appear to have a scant regard for runners or cyclists.

Swimming

This is first class cardiovascular exercise which utilizes almost every major muscle group in the body. In addition, since the body weight is adequately supported, it is ideal for those individuals who have problems with overweight or obesity or who may have orthopaedic or arthritic problems.

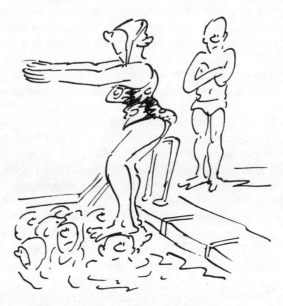

Since the body weight is supported by the water the constant jarring and shock which is a feature of running on hard roads is no longer a factor.

In general it is quite a social form of activity and is one in which it is easy to involve other members of the family. The disadvantage is obvious, i.e. you need to have ready access to a swimming pool. If you are fortunate enough to own your own then clearly you do not have a problem. However, for most of us access to a public baths is required and this obviously imposes certain restrictions. Even if this is convenient from a geographical point of view, there are other problems. Pools are often crowded with young children, especially during the school holidays and at weekends. This can make steady, good quality swimming hazardous, especially when you have to negotiate the diving board area. It tends also to be more time-consuming because apart from the exercise period, one also has to take into account travelling to and from the pool, plus changing time. However, if it is a form of exercise which you enjoy, and particularly if you are overweight or have arthritic or other joint problems, then it is, without doubt, an excellent choice.

Cycling

This is another superb cardiovascular exercise. Top class cyclists are probably the fittest cardiovascular athletes in the world. Cycling can be made as hard or as easy as you wish and it can be a solitary or a social activity. This flexibility makes it ideal in several respects. There are few more pleasant ways of taking your exercise than spinning along quiet country lanes on a balmy summer evening. Whether you ride for ten miles or 110 it is an enormously enjoyable form of exercise which is never boring.

The problem nowadays is that many roads are unsuitable for leisure cycling simply because of the sheer weight of traffic which they carry. The other problem, of course, is that in the winter months, when it becomes dark and cold and wet, it is even more dangerous, both from the point of view of other road users and also because of ice and snow. An alternative therefore is to use a stationary exercise bicycle.

The use of an exercise bicycle has a number of very significant advantages. Traffic is not a problem and you can choose any time of the day to exercise. Since it is essentially non-weight-bearing, it is ideal for the obese or for those with arthritic or other orthopaedic problems. In combination with the correct diet it substantially facilitates fairly rapid and sustained loss of body fat and we have a number of individuals who have lost as much as 40 lb using this form of exercise. It also has the advantage that since it is present in the home there is a high probability that other members of the family will also use it. An important advantage is that the intensity of exercise can be closely controlled because counting your pulse rate using this form of exercise is quite easy. If you are extremely unfit or obese then the use of a stationary exercise bicycle for two or three months prior to a running programme has considerable advantages.

The major disadvantage is that most people find sitting on an exercise bicycle and pedalling for 30 minutes exceedingly boring. The problem, however, is not insurmountable because there are simply ways and means by which you can occupy your mind during the exercise period; playing music, watching a television programme or even talking to others in the room are simple means of distraction. Many of the subjects who attend out laboratory opt to exercise during the evening news programme; this is 25 or 30 minutes long and therefore offers a warm-up and warm-down period and a 20-minute fairly intense activity period.

Exercise bicycles come in a wide variety of patterns and styles and there is an enormous range of quality. Some of them are frankly rubbish and it is extremely important that you buy the best quality machine you can afford; it will certainly pay dividends in the long run.

Squash

In recent years squash has become an extremely popular form of leisure-time activity. We are discussing it in detail here because we do not recommend it as a primary form of cardiovascular conditioning. The reasons for this will become evident later, but we would emphasize that it is not the game *per se* about which we have reservations, but rather the physical state of some of those who play it.

Squash attracts people from a very wide range of age groups and physical abilities. It is a highly demanding game which places a great strain on the cardiovascular system. It also imposes substantial demands upon the muscles and joints, as a consequence of which injuries to tendons and ligaments are common. However it is the isometric* component of squash together with the very high heart rates which are often induced that makes it potentially dangerous. Isometric exercise tends to produce higher blood pressures and since, as we have seen previously, the oxygen demand of the heart is proportional to the blood pressure multiplied by the heart rate (the rate–pressure product) it follows that the oxygen requirements of the heart are very substantially increased during squash. In a situation where the coronary arteries supplying that heart are normal then an increased coronary blood flow will provide the necessary oxygen requirements without difficulty. However, where the artery is significantly narrowed due to fatty plaque formation (atheroma), the heart may not be able to achieve the necessary blood and oxygen supply. This imblance between oxygen requirements and supply is potentially very dangerous. Since we also know that most men in middle life have evidence of arterial narrowing at least to some degree, and that some of them may have quite marked narrowing of their coronary arteries without any symptoms, it follows that squash cannot be a recommended form of cardiovascular conditioning. We know that the energy requirements of a hard squash game are considerable; perhaps rising to as much as 17 or 18 METs. In our experience many regular squash players have MET capacities of only 10 or 11 and are clearly not fit enough to play a game of that intensity.

From what has been said above, it is hardly surprising that many cases of sudden death and heart attack are reported to have occurred as a consequence of playing squash either during or shortly after the game. There are probably an equal number that go unreported.

We believe that squash is a game for young, fit individuals. For those over the age of 40 who wish to play there is a simple but extremely important rule of thumb – get fit to play squash, DO NOT PLAY SQUASH TO GET FIT. In other words, you require some other form of

---

* In pure isometric exercise both ends of the muscle are fixed and no movement occurs in the joint involved. An extreme example would be attempting to lift a colossal weight which you are simply incapable of lifting; for example, trying to lift a bar which was chained to the floor. If you are using a barbell then with a very light weight it is easy for you to contract your biceps, but as the weight increases, contracting the muscle becomes more difficult and the isometric component increases; at a point where the weight was so heavy that you simply could not flex your arm, the contraction of the muscle would be purely isometric.

cardiovascular fitness training prior to playing squash. Even then, the cardiovascular demands can be substantial. This is exacerbated by the fact that the game is, by its very nature, so highly competitive. This is, of course, part of its excitement, but we all know the syndrome – the man in his mid-fifties who is that most dangerous of all animals, the once-a-week squash player, who decides to challenge his son-in-law, who is 25 years younger, 40 lbs lighter and substantially fitter, to a match. After 10 or 15 minutes of this our 55-year-old is struggling. He is sweating heavily and beginning to look slightly pale or even grey. If he is wise he will stop at this point, but this hardly ever happens because if he had been wise, he would not have started playing in the first place. So he presses on regardless. In the heat of competition he may choose to ignore the pain in his chest or in his arm and because he ignores warning signs of this kind he is entering a new and extremely dangerous area. Squash is not alone in inducing this form of lemming-like behaviour, but the specific characteristics of the game make it especially likely.

It is simply a question of common sense. If you are fit and have no major medical problems, such as hypertension or marked obesity, then there is no reason why you should not play and enjoy what is a very exciting game. But, do not be tempted into trying to prove that you are every bit as good as you were 20 years ago. You are not. Your waistline may have already told you so, and the first two or three minutes of a squash game with a man half your age will probably confirm your worst suspicions. Play with people of a similar age and ability, and if you observe your partner in some difficulty, try to resist the temptation to try to finally 'wipe him out' – you just may succeed!

We are often told by some individuals that the fact that they are unfit and overweight does not really matter because they only play 'social squash'. We are not sure what this means, but if the implication is that this game is in some way non-competitive, then they clearly cannot be playing squash!

Badminton is an excellent alternative. It is still competitive but in general it does not impose anything like the cardiovascular demands which are a characteristic of squash. It is also a very social game, and many people find the social interaction of leisure activity extremely important.

In summary, squash is for those below the age of 50 with a normal blood pressure and a high aerobic capacity, who play regularly and who will also probably take part in other forms of cardiovascular exercise such as running or swimming.

It is clear from what we have said above that running/jogging, cycling (including the use of a stationary exercise bicycle) and swimming are excellent forms of exercise for cardiovascular conditioning. They are not the only ones of course, but in general they are the easiest to initiate and comply with. Each one has its own advantages and disadvantages and obviously it is up to the individual to make the choice which suits him best. Combinations of exercise are very good also since they tend to reduce boredom and therefore increase compliance. Remember that even if you play a sport such as football, rugby or netball etc., then in addition a regular cardiovascular conditioning exercise would be great benefit to you.

How Hard, How Long and How Often?

The intensity, duration and frequency of exercise are of crucial importance when discussing effective cardiovascular conditioning programmes. Many scientists have manipulated these three factors in an effort to identify which is the most effective in producing an increase in aerobic capacity (fitness). It is now evident that the changes produced by a training programme are directly related to the total work performed during that programme and are a direct extension of the frequency, intensity and duration of the training.

Intensity

Intensity is simply the rate of doing work. For example, if subject A runs five miles in 30 minutes, i.e. six minutes per mile, this would be a training session of lower intensity than subject B, who ran six miles in 30 minutes, i.e. five minutes per mile (this assumes, of course, that the aerobic capacity ($\dot{V}O_2$ max) of both individuals is approximately the same). Note in this example that the duration of the exercise was the same but the intensity was different. So we can see that the intensity is very important because it allows us to increase the total work performed whilst exercising for the same duration. As an extreme example, it is obvious that expending 300 calories during ten minutes' intense running will have very different cardiovascular and metabolic effects on the body than expending the same amount of calories during one hour's walking. So the intensity of exercise is a very important variable. The 30-minute session of your neighbour is not necessarily superior to your own 15-minute session, and it could be inferior if the total work performed was less.

Another method of assessing the intensity of exercise during your own training session is to express the exercise as a portion of the heart rate reserve. Your heart rate reserve is the difference between your heart rate in a relaxed, resting situation, and your age predicted maximum heart rate (APMHR). A key fact for consideration here is that your APMHR has nothing to do with how fit you are. Two individuals of the same age, one super-fit and the other extremely unfit, would have the same APMHRs. To assess your maximum heart rate you subtract your age from 220. (A 20-year-old would have an APMHR of 220 − 20 = 200, and a 40-year-old would have an APMHR of 180. This is only a rough approximation, but in practice if is usually sufficiently accurate. The maximum heart rate is that point at which the heart is simply unable to beat any faster.

Once you have established your APMHR you can calculate your heart rate reserve by subtracting your resting heart rate from your APMHR. Let us suppose that the 20-year-old and the 40-year-old man have the same resting heart rate, i.e. 60 beats per minute. The heart rate reserve for these two individuals would be 140 and 120 respectively, i.e. for the 20-year-old, 200 − 60 = 140, and for the 40-year-old 180 − 60 = 120.

To calculate appropriate heart rates for a cardiovascular training effect during exercise, the following calculation is required: training heart rate = 60–90 per cent of heart rate reserve + resting heart rate. Exercise intensities of between 60 and 90 per cent have been recommended to gain improvement in performance. We shall illustrate the calculations for the 20-year-old and the 40-year-old respectively to show how we arrive at the appropriate heart rate intensity for exercise. We shall be assuming that we wish to exercise at a 75 per cent intensity.

In the case of the 20-year-old the APMHR was 220 − 20 = 200. The heart rate reserve, assuming a resting heart rate of 60 was 200 − 60 = 140. So the exercise heart rate is given by 140 × 0.75 + 60 = 165. The appropriate heart rate for a training effect is thus 165 beats per minute. For the 40-year-old we calculate the training heart rate as follows: APMHR was 220 − 40 = 180. The heart rate reserve, assuming a resting heart rate of 60, was 180 − 60 = 120. Thus, 120 × 0.75 + 60 = 150. So in this case the appropriate heart rate for a training effect is 150 beats per minute.

To summarize, to calculate the intensity of exercise in terms of pulse rate, take the following steps:

1 Calculate the APMHR by subtracting your age from 220.
2 Calculate the heart rate reserve by subtracting the resting heart rate from APMHR.
3 Take 75 per cent of the heart rate reserve, i.e. heart rate reserve × 0.75, and then add the resting heart rate.

The reader should now be able to calculate his or her own training heart rate according to the steps outlined above. A good training intensity to aim for is 75 per cent. A simple and quick means of assessing the appropriate heart rate range for exercise is illustrated in appendix 3.

Frequency and Duration

Most people contemplating exercise programmes are very concerned about the number of times per week that they will have to exercise. They are also concerned that it may take up a substantial amount of time. Evidence clearly suggests that three or four exercise sessions per week of 30 minutes' duration will suffice. Three sessions of 20 minutes of good quality exercise is probably adequate to maintain an acceptable, although minimal, level of cardiovascular conditioning. However, like all good things in life, the more you invest the more you gain. We would remind you that research tells us that training benefits are directly related to the total work performed. If two individuals were engaged in exercise by running six miles in 30 minutes then the mode and the intensity of their programmes would be the same. However, if one of these individuals was exercising three times per week and the other five times per week, then the total work performed by the latter would be greater and therefore the post-training improvement in performance would be greater.

We must bear in mind, however, that improved performance is not necessarily the goal. We are primarily seeking to encourage individuals to perform sufficient exercise to maintain health. The requirements for this, as stated, are three or four 20- or 30-minute sessions per week, at an intensity related to 75 per cent of heart rate reserve. Clearly, if performance is the prime goal then the requirements both in terms of frequency, duration and intensity will be very much higher. Running a marathon in under 2 hours and 30 minutes will require a very substantial commitment in terms of time and effort, but this is not the aim for most of us.

We must all the time consider the total work performed. If two individuals who are using their heart rates to guide them, as previously described, are both exercising for 30 minutes at 75 per cent of their heart rate reserve, then the five times a week runner will obviously be doing more physiological work than the three times a week runner and would therefore be expected to make greater gains in work capacity. In some short training studies of eight to ten weeks, the group of five-day-per-week trainers showed greater gains in work performance than the three-days-per-week trainers. However, when the three-day trainers continued to train for a further five weeks. thus equalling the work performed by the five-day group, the work capacity of the two groups was similar. Thus the total work performed during a training programme can be achieved by a multiplicity of changes in the intensity, duration and frequency of exercise. These programmes, although differing in many respects, can be equally effective in bringing about an improvement in work capacity and a readiness to perform exercise. Training at 60 per cent of the heart rate reserve on only one or two occasions a week for 15 minutes will obviously not produce anything like the same results as training at 85 per cent of the heart rate reserve for 30 minutes on five occasions.

To summarize: the improvement in fitness (readiness for living) is a function of the total work performed which in turn is a function of frequency, duration and intensity. We recommend as a useful guide that to produce a significant training effect the individual should exercise for three or four 30-minute sessions per week based on a target heart rate of 75 per cent of the heart rate reserve. Some people would probably prefer a greater intensity of exercise with a shorter duration, for example 15 minutes using 80–90 per cent of heart rate reserve. While this may be acceptable for younger or fit individuals, this is certainly not the type of regimen we would recommend for the over-40, first-time exerciser. A longer duration with a lower intensity (perhaps 60–75 per cent) for perhaps half to three-quarters of an hour on three to four occasions per week would be safe and effective. If sometimes you are unable to perform three sessions per week, then one or two will suffice and this will not have a major influence on your fitness capacity. There is some evidence that once a reasonable standard of fitness has been achieved, two 30-minute sessions of exercise per week are sufficient to maintain this level of fitness.

Bear in mind, however, that activity patterns, even of high intensity, which are only carried out on one occasion per week, or less, do not bring about a significant training effect. More importantly, because physiological improvements are not obtained in the once-a-week exerciser, these exercising habits can be dangerous, especially in the over-40-year-old male. Examples of this form of irregular (low frequency) exercise habit are the occasional game of squash or five-a-side soccer or basketball, all involving keen competition. These forms of exercise inevitably bring together groups of people with differing ages and physical work capacity. It is quite possible for a 20-year-old, reasonably fit individual, to be casually involved in a 30-minute game of five-a-side soccer which may demand only 50–60 per cent of his maximum aerobic capacity, while at the same time his 45-year-old, obese and mildly hypertensive boss, equipped with the inevitable Type A personality, is wheezing and gasping his way through the same game which is demanding 90 per cent of his maximum aerobic capacity.

Again we see a dangerous difference in the readiness to perform between two people who are competing against each other. In addition, because the frequency of these games is low, there is no conditioning effect and therefore each game represents a renewed trauma on the physiological systems. These forms of infrequent, competitive, high intensity exercise represent all that is bad about a leisure-time activity. Many of the sudden deaths which feature in the press are the results of badly prescribed exercise, but unfortunately this is never highlighted and the wise exerciser is made to feel unnecessarily apprehensive on his pleasant, sensibly designed, morning run.

Gently Does It

Getting Started

We believe that all cardiovascular exercise should be preceded by an effective warm-up programme. This should be designed to passively stretch muscles and joints through a whole range of movement and to stimulate the cardiovascular system by very low level, rhythmical work to a heart rate of about 100 beats per minute. In addition, a period of 'warm' down is of paramount important, with particular awareness to prevention of blood pooling in the lower extremities. During exercise the oxygen requirements of the muscles are such that there is a tremendous increase in blood flow. An abrupt cessation of vigorous exercise results in substantial 'pooling' of blood due to the fact that when the muscles are contracting they return blood to the heart in a highly efficient manner. When exercise is discontinued suddenly, this pooling effect may result in a feeling of light headedness or even fainting. It follows that a five- or ten-minute warm-down by walking is a very wise habit, and one which you should always put into practice. It is important to remember that regardless of the type of mode of exercise you choose, a warm-up and warm-down are essential.

In addition to the cardiovascular development, we believe that an all-round conditioning programme is wise and we also recommend that flexibility and strength should be components of your training programme. Unfortunately the development of strength with safety requires special apparatus and it also demands a lot of time. It usually necessitates joining a local health studio or weight training club and you should try to ensure you receive instruction from somebody who is competent to provide it. However, flexibility can be comfortably absorbed into a cardiovascular conditioning programme and many of the exercises to stretch key muscles and joints can become a very valuable part of a warm-up and warm-down routine.

In appendix 4 we have demonstrated several flexibility exercises that are ideal for the pre-run warm-up. If you get into an organized routine you will remember them with ease and run through them smoothly. All warm-up exercises must be carried out passively, i.e. you should be able to stop the muscle movement at any time. There should be no forcing or sudden jerking of the movement. You should gently stretch the muscle to the point of limitation by carefully applied pressure. So-called ballistic movements, characterized by rapid jerking and swinging, are unwise and can sometimes have the opposite effect, for rather than lengthening the muscle these movements may actually shorten it by stimulating the short receptors that tend to counteract violent forms of stretching.

Start your exercises with the lower leg muscles, move up to the upper leg muscles, the hips, the abdomen, the lower and upper back, shoulders and neck. Each exercise selected should be executed ten times (ten repetitions) and each group of ten repetitions should be repeated three times (i.e. three sets of ten repetitions). Three sets of ten repetitions should bring about a pleasant perspiration and a heart rate of about 100 beats per minute in preparation for the main part of the cardiovascular exercise.

One final point is worthy of note. Whatever exercise you decide to do, you must learn to discriminate between genuinely feeling unwell and not being up to your exercise schedule, and being lazy. If you honestly do not feel like doing the exercise then the simple advice is to give it a miss. If you start the exercise and begin to find it extremely unpleasant, then you should discontinue it and leave it for another time. Most of us have good days and bad days and most of the days are indifferent. If you have a bad day, leave it. One or two missed training sessions will have virtually no effect on your overall fitness.

A little practical description of how to get started with your exercise would seem appropriate. We have chosen running/walking as the example here, but the principles apply equally to other forms of exercise. Following your warm-up, which can take place indoors or outdoors depending upon the weather, you are now ready for your first 30 minutes of running. Remember, however, that this is your first run. The intention is to gently jog/walk for 15 minutes from the start, to turn around and jog/walk back for 15 minutes. This may sound easy, but to undertake this task if you have been entirely sedentary for some time will take patience and time. If we assume that you are 40-years-old, we know from our previous discussion that your heart rate reserve is 120 beats per minute (assuming a resting heart rate of 60 beats per minute). If we assume that you are to run at 75 per cent of your capacity, your target heart rate during exercise will be 150 beats per minute.

Taking the Pulse

At this point we need to consider how you should go about taking your own pulse in order to control the intensity of the exercise. There are two places in which the pulse can be taken without difficulty – the radial pulse and the carotid pulse. To take the radial pulse turn your right hand palm upwards and with the fingers of the left hand gently feel the pulse on the outer aspect of the wrist (figure 7.1). To take the carotid pulse you should

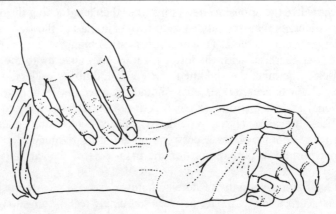

Figure 7.1 Taking the radial pulse.

first feel the Adams apple (cricoid cartilage) in the front of the neck. Move your fingers to approximately one to one and a half inches either side of this and you will feel the carotid pulse. Never compress both carotid pulses at once. The procedure for taking the carotid pulse correctly is shown in figure 7.2.

To count the pulse you should count the number of beats over ten seconds and multiply the answer by six. If you try to count the pulse for any longer than this the pulse rate begins to fall off and you will obtain a false impression of the intensity of exercise which you have just performed. If you decide that your target heart rate during exercise is 150

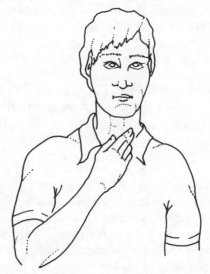

Figure 7.2 Taking the carotid pulse.

beats per minute, then you should aim to count 25 beats over ten seconds. If your target heart rate is 160 beats per minute, then a ten-second count should give you 26–27 beats.

Returning to our 40-year-old with a target heart rate of 150 beats per minute, the ten-second count should be 25. The aim therefore is to walk/run with the heart beating at approximately this number of beats. So, start to run gently and when you begin to feel breathless walk for a few seconds and check your pulse. If the ten-second count is 20 beats you can work a little harder during the running phase. If it is 30 beats then you should reduce the intensity of the running phase. If the pulse is approximately 25, intensity of exercise is correct. In general a good guide is that at the correct level of exertion you should be able to hold a conversation with someone without too much difficulty. As you are taking your pulse it is important to think about how you feel at that point. Do you feel good or do you feel uncomfortable? See if you can predict your heart rate just before you take it, i.e., learn to perceive your own exertion accurately. With a little practice you will be able to perceive the intensity of your exercise with considerable accuracy, even to within two or three beats per minute. With experience your perception of your exertion will become so good that you will no longer need to take your pulse as a routine procedure.

As time goes on you will need to walk less and you will be able to run more. For the first session you may only be able to run for a few yards and it may take you several weeks to be able to run any appreciable distance without walking. This is a temporary state and you should not be discouraged. Improvements will come, provided you persevere. If you keep to the heart rates which have been suggested then a cardiovascular conditioning effect will occur within a relatively short period of time. Patience and perseverance are the key words here.

After a variable period, which will depend upon your initial physical state, you will be able to run for 15 minutes out and 15 minutes back without stopping. Clearly as your fitness or 'readiness to perform' improves, you will be able to run a longer distance in the same period of time. Remember, however, that it is the time that matters as much as the intensity and so although your fitness is improving you should continue to run for 30 minutes. Do not make the mistake of rushing out on your first day and trying to cover six miles. This will do your cardiovascular system no good at all and will probably result in considerable muscle soreness so that you will be unable to run – or perhaps even walk properly – for the next week.

A few months into your exercise programme you will have the exhilaration of being able to run for 30 minutes non-stop and eventually you will be able to run for substantially longer if you so wish. Now that you have become fit, and assuming that you are healthy, you need not pay any great

Table 7.1 Predicted aerobic fitness classification: men

Category	Measure	Age (years)			
		Under 30	30–39	40–49	50+
Poor	12 min distance (miles)	1.0–1.24	0.95–1.14	0.85–1.04	0.80–0.99
	1.5 mile time (min:sec)	14:31–16:30	15:31–17:30	16:31–18:30	17:01–19:00
	Predicted oxygen uptake (VO_2 max ml kg^{-1} min^{-1})	25.0–33.7	24.7–30.1	24.6–26.4	24.5–24.9
Fair	12 min. distance (miles)	1.25–1.49	1.15–1.39	1.05–1.29	1.0–1.24
	1.5 mile time (min:sec)	12:01–14:30	13:01–15:30	14:01–16:30	14:31–17:00
	Predicted oxygen uptake (VO_2 max ml kg^{-1} min^{-1})	33.8–42.5	30.2–39.1	26.5–35.4	25.0–33.7
Good	12 min. distance (miles)	1.50–1.74	1.40–1.64	1.30–1.54	1.25–1.49
	1.5 mile time (min:sec)	10:16–12:00	11:01–13:00	11:31–14:00	12:01–14:30
	Predicted oxygen uptake (VO_2 max ml kg^{-1} min^{-1})	42.6–51.5	39.2–47.9	35.5–44.4	33.8–42.5
Excellent	12 min. distance (miles)	1.75–2.00	1.65–1.90	1.55–1.80	1.50–1.75
	1.5 mile time (min:sec)	8:45–10:15	9:30–11:00	10:00–11:30	10:30–12:00
	Predicted oxygen uptake (VO_2 max ml kg^{-1} min^{-1})	51.6–60.2	48.0–57.0	44.5–53.6	42.6–51.6
Superior	12 min. distance (miles)	2.00+	1.90+	1.80+	1.75+
	1.5 mile time (min:sec)	<8:45	<9:30	<10:00	<10:30
	Predicted oxygen uptake (VO_2 max ml kg^{-1} min^{-1})	60.2+	57.0+	53.6+	51.6+

Table 7.2 Predicted aerobic fitness classification: women

Category	Measure	Age (years)			
		Under 30	30–39	40–49	50+
Poor	12 min distance (miles)	0.95–1.14	0.85–1.04	0.75–0.94	0.65–0.84
	1.5 mile time (min:sec)	15:31–17:30	16:31–18:30	17:32–19:30	18:31–20:30
	Predicted oxygen uptake (VO_2 max ml kg^{-1} min^{-1})	23.6–30.1	23.5–29.4	23.4–28.9	23.3–27.0
Fair	12 min. distance (miles)	1.15–1.34	1.05–1.24	0.95–1.14	0.85–1.04
	1.5 mile time (min:sec)	13:01–15:30	14:01–16:30	15:01–17:30	16:31–18:30
	Predicted oxygen uptake (VO_2 max ml kg^{-1} min^{-1})	30.2–37.0	29.5–35.8	29.0–35.0	27.1–33.0
Good	12 min. distance (miles)	1.35–1.64	1.25–1.54	1.15–1.44	1.05–1.34
	1.5 mile time (min:sec)	11:16–13:00	12:01–14:00	12:31–15:00	13:31–16:30
	Predicted oxygen uptake (VO_2 max ml kg^{-1} min^{-1})	37.1–47.9	35.9–45.0	35.1–40.9	33.1–37.0
Excellent	12 min. distance (miles)	1.65–1.85	1.55–1.75	1.45–1.65	1.35–1.55
	1.5 mile time (min:sec)	9:45–11:15	10:30–12:00	11:00–12:30	12:00–13:30
	Predicted oxygen uptake (VO_2 max ml kg^{-1} min^{-1})	48.0–55.2	45.1–51.6	41.0–48.0	37.1–44.6
Superior	12 min. distance (miles)	1.85+	1.75+	1.65+	1.55+
	1.5 mile time (min:sec)	<9:45	<10:30	<11:00	<12:00
	Predicted oxygen uptake (VO_2 max ml kg^{-1} min^{-1})	55.2+	51.6+	48.0+	44.6+

attention to target heart rates during exercise. Your perception of your own intensity of exercise will be so good that you can run the 'engine' at remarkably precise levels. If you feel strong then there is no reason why you should not, occasionally, push yourself a little harder. However, you should never push yourself to the limits of your capacity as it places an unnecessary strain on your system and there is no evidence that exercising to the point of exhaustion will do you any good. Remember you are supposed to be enjoying it and if it becomes unpleasant or painful you should reduce the workload. Do not be tempted into believing that unless it is hurting it cannot be doing you any good. Although this is advice often given it is complete nonsense.

Assessing Your Progress

The most precise way of assessing your improved cardiovascular efficiency is to undergo a direct measurement of your maximum oxygen consumption ($\dot{V}O_2$ max) in a laboratory environment. It is unfortunate that these measurements require sophisticated technology and their interpretation also requires a high level of expertise. You can, however, obtain an approximate guide to your $\dot{V}O_2$ max by referring to tables 7.1 and 7.2. They relate to the distance you can run or run/walk in 12 minutes and the time it takes you to run a measured 1.5 miles. An approximate estimate from these two parameters gives your aerobic capacity ($\dot{V}O_2$ max). The figures in the tables take age into account.

Most sedentary individuals who attend our laboratory have a maximum oxygen consumption of $35-40$ ml kg^{-1} min^{-1}. A more active individual who is perhaps exercising for two or three 30-minute sessions per week may have a $\dot{V}O_2$ max of $45-50$ ml kg^{-1} min^{-1}. In a good class club athlete it will be 70 or more and in a world class athlete, 90 or above. You will need to bear in mind that these capacities are to a large extent genetically endowed. In other words, without question, you cannot become a great athlete, you have to be born one. Nevertheless, even if your aerobic capacity is only modest it can usually be improved by at least $15-20$ per cent and you can substantially improved your readiness for living. A $\dot{V}O_2$ max of 90 ml kg^{-1} min^{-1} or above represents an extraordinary high level of cardiovascular efficiency and testing a world class athlete with this capacity serves only to emphasize the enormous spectrum of ability in any given population.

8

Applying the Principles

In preceding chapters we have outlined in some detail how to identify and manipulate various coronary risk factors, how to exercise and thus how to acquire a 'readiness for living'.

In this chapter we shall briefly illustrate the practical application of these principles by discussing a number of case histories. We shall also show how a prescribed programme of exercise can be applied to benefit those who have already developed heart disease and suffered a heart attack.

Case Histories

The individuals whose case histories are presented here have all attended our own laboratory and have been chosen because they are an accurate representation of the large number of individuals who have attended our department during the past five to ten years. All these subjects were entirely symptom-free on presentation, with no history of cardiac disease. The reader should bear in mind that we are only including the laboratory data that are directly relevant to the discussion and that the recommendations given are only summarized briefly here. Nevertheless, these histories do serve to illustrate adequately the application of the principles we have discussed.

Case 1 – a 55-year-old Businessman

He was entirely symptom free, although there was some family history of note in that both his mother and his father had suffered with coronary heart disease before the age of 65. His father had died at the age of 52 from a heart attack and his mother was being treated for angina.

Initial assessment revealed a weight of 100 kg; we estimated his body fat percentage at 32 per cent. His resting blood pressure was marginally elevated at 150/100 mmHg. He was entirely sedentary and paid no specific attention to his diet. This was subsequently reflected in a blood cholesterol of 9 mmol/l and a maximum oxygen consumption ($\dot{V}O_2$ max) of only 34 ml kg^{-1} min^{-1}. He also admitted to smoking 30 cigarettes a day. The exercise electrocardiograph was entirely within normal limits.

Recommendations

This man had the following risk factors:

1 A significant family history of coronary heart disease.
2 Elevated blood cholesterol.
3 Inactivity.
4 Obesity (although we actually estimated his body fat percentage, he would have been classified as obese according to the Royal College of Physicians classification outlined previously).
5 Borderline essential hypertension.
6 Smoking.

The family history was obviously a risk factor which was not amenable to correction. The remaining risk factors were dealt with in the following way.

First, he was advised to reduce his salt intake substantially in order to help to control his borderline essential hypertension. This, in combination with weight loss of 20 lb, subsequently reduced his blood pressure to within normal limits. His estimated body fat percentage fell from 30 to 24 per cent. In the first instance we recommended the use of a stationary exercise bicycle, although when he had lost weight he was able to take up a running programme successfully. This resulted in a substantial improvement in his $\dot{V}O_2$ max from 34 ml to 53 ml kg^{-1} min^{-1}. A low fat, high fibre diet, which he used in combination with his regular exercise programme, not only facilitated the weight loss that we recommended but also resulted in a very substantial reduction in his blood cholesterol from 9 mmol/l to 5.8 mmol/l. Since the exercise also result in an increase in HDL from 1 to 1.4 mmol/l, the coronary heart disease risk ratio (i.e. the total cholesterol divided by the HDL cholesterol) fell from 9 to 4.1; this was clearly a major improvement. Finally he was able to discontinue cigarette smoking completely.

Case 2 – a 40-year-old Housewife

This lady was sedentary and obese (estimated body fat of 35 per cent). She had been trying for a number of years to achieve and maintain adequate weight loss but had been unsuccessful. She had given up smoking approximately five years earlier. There was some relevant family history of cardiac disease in that both her parents had suffered heart attacks in their mid-50s. Her own previous medical and surgical history was unremarkable apart from a history of lower back problems (lumbo-sacral disc prolapse). The resting blood pressure was 110/70 mmHg and her blood cholesterol was found to be elevated at 11 mmol/l. It is also relevant that her husband apparently suffered a heart attack at the age of 42 and was subsequently found to have a blood cholesterol level of 9 mmol/l. The couple had two children, aged 15 and 17. Her functional assessment revealed a $\dot{V}O_2$ max of only 25 ml kg $^{-1}$ min $^{-1}$, indicating a low aerobic capacity.

Recommendations

The family history was obviously relevant in that it served to enhance the importance of the enthusiastic manipulation of those factors which were potentially amenable to change. Her obesity was a major problem but she subsequently lost 25 lb, utilizing a stationary exercise bicycle and exercising at the appropriate intensity, frequency and duration in combination with a low fat diet to achieve the necessary weight loss over a period of six months. A stationary exercise bicycle was recommended because of the non-weight bearing nature of the exercise and the fact that she was known to have a history of lower back problems. Her blood cholesterol responded well to dietary manipulation and eventually fell to 6.5 mmol/l. As a result of her weight loss and cardiovascular training programme, her $\dot{V}O_2$ max increased to a respectable 40 ml kg^{-1} min^{-1}. In view of the family history, both her children were screened and both had blood cholesterol levels above 6 mmol/l; these subsequently responded adequately to appropriate dietary therapy.

Case 3 – a 38-year-old Policeman

There was no strong family history of coronary heart disease and he himself was entirely symptom-free. He played squash occasionally, usually two or three times per month, but took nothing else in the way of regular exercise. He smoked 20 cigarettes a day. His blood pressure was normal at 130/70 mmHg and he did not have any substantial weight problem since his estimated body fat percentage was 20 per cent. His maximum oxygen consumption on direct measurement was 43 ml kg^{-1} min^{-1} and this represented a MET capacity of just over 12. The blood cholesterol was acceptable at 5.5 mmol/l.

Recommendations

The two major risk factors in this case were the fact that he was essentially sedentary and also a heavy smoker. The fact that he was an 'occasional' squash player was also a little worrying. We recommended he should discontinue cigarette smoking and certainly improve his rather poor cardiovascular capacity with the appropriate conditioning programme. He subsequently took up running and swimming and improved his $\dot{V}O_2$ max to 56 ml kg^{-1} min^{-1}. This represented a measured improvement in his functional capacity and improved his MET capacity to 16. This gave him a sufficient standard of cardiovascular fitness to be able to play a very effective and safe game of squash. After some difficulty he did manage to cease cigarette smoking completely.

Case 4 – a 48-year-old Senior Banker

There was no strong family history of cardiac disease and his own previous medical and surgical history was unremarkable. When he originally attended the laboratory his body fat was estimated at 35 per cent and his weight was 91.5 kg. His resting blood pressure was 148/88 mmHg. On direct testing his $\dot{V}O_2$ max was 36.6 ml kg^{-1} min^{-1}. Subsequent evaluation of his blood lipids revealed a blood cholesterol of 6.5 mmol/l and an HDL cholesterol of 1.48 mmol/l. His coronary heart disease risk ratio was therefore slightly below average at 4.5. He was a non-smoker.

Recommendations

It was suggested that he should utilize a low fat, high fibre diet and commence a running programme. This he subsequently did and during the next six to nine months he made a tremendous improvement in his overall risk factor profile. His body weight reduced from 91.5 kg to 79 kg and his body fat percentage dropped from 35 to 27 per cent. This represents a weight loss of almost 30 lb. The resting blood pressure dropped to 138/70 mmHg and on functional assessment his $\dot{V}O_2$ max increased from 36.6 ml kg^{-1} min^{-1} to 53 ml kg^{-1} min^{-1}. This obviously represents a major improvement in his cardiorespiratory capacity. The blood cholesterol fell from 6.56 mmol/l to 5.17 mmol/l and the HDL cholesterol increased to 1.94 mmol/l. This gave him an excellent coronary heart disease risk ratio at 2.7. He continues to improve and now has a first class standard of cardiovascular fitness.

Case 5 – a 52-year-old Solicitor

This gentleman had been physically active all his life and there was no significant family history of note. He ran regularly and had done so since he was 14 years old. His resting blood pressure was normal at 110/70 mmHg. His blood cholesterol was 5.4 mmol/l. He was a non-smoker and in fact had never smoked in his life. He drank moderately and paid close attention to his diet. His functional capacity was measured directly and he had a $\dot{V}O_2$ max of 59 ml kg^{-1} min^{-1}, which places him easily in the 'excellent' category.

Recommendations

This man's coronary risk ratio was very low indeed and no specific recommendations were required, other than to continue to maintain his high levels of physical activity and to continue his interest in diet.

Case 6 – 29-year-old World Class Marathon Runner

This man is an elite athlete and runs approximately 100 miles per week. He had no family history of note and his resting blood pressure was normal at 120/68 mmHg. His blood cholesterol was 4.73 mmol/l. His estimated body fat was 8.5 per cent and his functional capacity was measured directly at 86.4 ml kg^{-1} min^{-1}. He paid close attention to his diet, utilizing a low fat, high fibre, high carbohydrate regime. He clearly needed to have adequate carbohydrate intake to fuel his exercise programme, since the muscles needed constantly replenishing with adequate glycogen.

Recommendations
Carry on!

The above brief examples illustrate how to apply the principles we have discussed in specific situations. You should now be in a position to do exactly the same thing and when you have dealt with the manipulation of any obvious coronary risk factors which you may have, you will then be able to plan your own training schedule in terms of frequency, duration and intensity, as outlined above.

Exercise Following a Heart Attack

There are a substantial number of individuals in our society who have already been unfortunate enough to develop coronary heart disease. For the majority of angina patients and those who have suffered a coronary thrombosis (post-coronary patients), we advocate a positive, enthusiastic approach to the problem. Although attitudes toward patients who have suffered heart attacks are now much more liberal, there is still a great deal of misunderstanding about the disease. Many people tend to ostracize post-coronary patients and regard them with a great deal of apprehension. The patients themselves lose confidence and personal esteem and the social effects on the family can be catastrophic.

It is interesting to note how opinions have changed over the last 50 years when considering the acute and long-term treatment of the post-coronary patient. In the 1930s strict procedures ensured limited movement during the hospital stay. Following discharge from hospital the patients must have felt totally helpless and forlorn as all forms of exercise and activity were forbidden for at least one year. The return to work was usually many months away and the morale and quality of life were extremely low. In the 1940s the ill-effects of bed rest were recognized, suspicions that were endorsed by the work of Soltein and co-workers in 1968. The current trend towards early mobilization probably started in Boston in the 1940s, with the chair treatment of Samuel Levine. This was based on the theory that sitting in a chair would increase the pooling of blood in the lower limbs and would decrease the amount of blood returning to the heart, resulting in a reduced cardiac workload. This routine of sitting in a chair for two hours per day from the first day following a heart attack reduced the likelihood of venous clotting, reduced the complications and decreased cardiac neurosis.

Since Levine's success with the early movement programme, a large proportion of the patients who have uncomplicated heart attacks undergo early 'in hospital' exercise, designed to prevent the deterioration of the cardiovascular system that is a feature of prolonged bed rest. These exercises are obviously of a low level of intensity and are individually prescribed and supervised by hospital personnel. The programme consists of calisthenics to increase flexibility and muscle strength and most self-care activities, such as shaving, feeding and bathing. The majority of patients leave hospital 10–14 days after the heart attack.

The home phase of rehabilitation is the period of most concern. It is a time of frustration and anxiety, with very poor direction. The patient has spent 10–14 days in hospital very closely monitored and develops a sense of dependency on the informed medical team who are a feature of his daily life. Quite suddenly he is surrounded by a loving family who are not very well informed, are lacking in confidence and feeling very apprehensive about their charge. When in doubt families tend to err on the side of caution, and restrictions and inhibitions become the order of the day. The usual advice given to the patient by the doctor is to walk twice daily within the limits of pain and most families become very concerned about this. Individuals within the family go out of their way to ensure that the patient's involvement in activities around the house is at a minimum. This increases frustration even further and can be the cause of considerable stress for both the patient and the family.

There are very few post-coronary rehabilitation programmes in Britain and those that are available are usually hospital-based. Patients do not like long associations with hospitals and therefore rehabilitation programmes that take place in a hospital environment usually have a poor compliance.

There is a need for rehabilitation programmes to be centered in many of the leisure facilities throughout the country. We would like to see one-year programmes of post-coronary rehabilitation started in hospitals but extending to recreational facilities within the area. With the increasing number of coronary artery bypass operations being performed there is also a need to include these patients within rehabilitation programmes. The evidence suggests that this group of patients will do particularly well on structured rehabilitation programmes. After one year's rehabilitation, post-coronary and post-bypass patients will usually have the confidence to continue and maintain a programme of exercise for life.

The goal of successful rehabilitation is to return the patient to the maximum achievable level of physical and psychological activity. The evidence suggests that structured exercise programmes not only improve the quality of life but, because they result in an increase in the functional capacity of the patient, they may well be protective against further heart attacks. This must be a very strong argument for post-coronary exercise. If we can increase the maximum energy capacity of the post-coronary patient, then all the everyday energy expenditure associated with work and leisure will put less strain on the system.

The energy costs of various activities, as we have seen, can be defined in metabolic units (METs). One MET is the energy expended per kilogramme of body weight, per minute when an average-sized man is resting in the sitting or lying position. By the time a coronary patient leaves hospital, his or her energy capacity ranges between 3 and 5 METs; this is low compared with the 10 MET capacity of a healthy sedentary man or the 20 MET capacity of the highly trained athlete. With a daily walking programme for two months the energy capacity can be raised from 5 to 7 METs. This energy capacity would in fact cover most of the less strenuous daily activities, but many leisure activities such as gardening (digging), badminton, jogging etc. would be well beyond the patient at this stage.

If the patient were now to embark upon an organized 12-month programme of medically supervised exercise, the MET capacity would increase to approximately 7–12 METs, resulting in a substantial improvement in the quality of life. A functional capacity of this order would enable the individual to carry out most daily work and leisure activities quite comfortably. The mountain walk, casual jog, non-competitive game of badminton and most gardening activities would be well within his capacity. Surely this must be the aim of most coronary patients.

Many physicians and general practitioners still share considerable concern about the dangers associated with exercise in the post-coronary patient. We believe, however, that the risks are minimal, provided that the programme of exercise is correctly prescribed and that the patients are totally informed about what is required of them.

One of the better rehabilitation programmes in Britain is the one centered at Preston in Lancashire. This programme is an excellent example of a community's combining the talents of scientists, educationalists and medical practitioners.

The Preston post-coronary patients embark upon an in-hospital rehabilitation programme commencing the day after admission to intensive care. The exercises are graduated and individually prescribed with cardiovascular responses being very carefully monitored. The patients who have no complications are usually discharged within 10–14 days after the heart attack. At three weeks post-coronary they return to the hospital where they undergo a functional exercise stress test. The stress test, in addition to assisting with prognosis, also provides valuable individual data which can be used to prescribe safe activity levels during the next stage of rehabilitation. In addition to the daily walking programme which is a feature of most coronary rehabilitation, Preston patients are encouraged to attend the occupational therapy unit in the hospital, to experience a variety of occupational activities designed to improve energy capacity and everyday competence.

At two months post-coronary the patients enter the third phase of their rehabilitation. Prior to entry all patients undergo a functional graded exercise stress test which consists of walking on a treadmill designed to assess the functional capacity of each patient. This provides the medical director with the necessary data to prescribe an individual exercise programme for each patient. The exercise stress test is a critical feature of post-coronary rehabilitation; in many instances it provides key information which enables the medical director to decide whether patients should be treated medically or surgically and it identifies many patients who would *not* benefit from an exercise programme.

For those patients who successfully complete the exercise stress test, a programme of exercise is designed on an individual basis, taking into account the patient's cardiovascular responses during exercise on the treadmill. The third phase of the rehabilitation is anticipated to last approximately one year. Evening exercise sessions are held in a sports hall in the centre of Preston three times per week. Each session lasts about one hour. A minimum attendance of two sessions per week is required. Each session is medically supervised by one of a team of general practitioners from the Preston area and the exercises are prescribed by individuals from a team of physiotherapists and physical educationalists. This is an excellent example of a range of specialists combining to provide a valuable service.

The exercise sessions consist of 15 minutes calisthenics, 15 minutes of running and 15 minutes of a selected recreation such as badminton, table tennis or volley ball. Each session is preceded by a five-minute warm-up and followed by a five minute warm-down. Patients have their own target heart rates which are converted, for ease of counting, to a ten-second count. Each patient is taught how to take his pulse accurately. This is critical because it enables the individual to assess objectively the intensity of the exercise which he is undergoing. For instance, if he were involved in a weekend ramble and a rather steep slope seemed difficult, a quick pulse assessment would enable him to decide whether he was over-perceiving his effort, or whether the pace of ascent was too intense and he would be wise to slow down. On no account should patients be encouraged to allow their heart rate to go above the target prescribed.

This method provides a post-coronary patient with a safe means of becoming involved in individually prescribed exercise designed to provide an energy expenditure of approximately 1,000 kcal per week, which is the threshold required to bring about cardiovascular improvement. Patients are re-tested at 6, 9 and 12 months. At the completion of the third phase all patients are encouraged to embark on a non-supervised maintenance programme, designed to ensure that they maintain life-long fitness.

The Preston programme has been running for eight years and the rate of deaths and re-infarctions (further heart attacks) in this group of patients is lower when comparisons are made with sedentary post-coronary patients in other parts of the country, although the numbers are, as yet, too small for statistical conclusions. What *can* be said with absolute confidence at the moment is that none of the patients on the programme have died during the stress testing or whilst exercising. The programme has clearly established, in conjunction with many of the American programmes, that exercise prescription for post-coronary patients is a safe procedure.

Unfortunately, Britain is sadly lacking in the provision of programmes of rehabilitation for the post-coronary patient. We should be seeking a position at least on a par with that in North America and indeed some European countries. Whilst we wait for developments in this area, many patients are doomed to apprehension and neurosis. They tend to underestimate their true capacities and continue with a sedentary lifestyle which is more inactive than the one they had prior to their heart attack. This in turn makes them prone to further problems. In addition, smoking, obesity, high blood pressure, stress etc. may then be superimposed on an already damaged heart and the prognosis for these patients is obviously not good.

We cannot wait until programmes such as the one at Preston are adequately distributed across the country. At this moment many patients would gain substantial benefits from a carefully prescribed programme of exercise. We believe that during the first six months, post-coronary patients should ideally exercise under medical supervision. Having said that,we also believe that providing the exercise prescription takes into account the absence of medical supervision, and increases the safety margin to allow for this, a large proportion of post-coronary patients could embark on a home-based programme without undue risk. From our experience with early coronary patients, perception of cardiac effort can be sadly misleading. We would argue that all post-coronary patients should undergo a functional exercise stress test and that a home-based programme could then be safely precribed on the basis of this test. We recognize the dangers inherent in exercising post-coronary patients and accept that there is no fool-proof method. There are documented instances of patients who have been prescribed exercise following a stress test experiencing serious problems. We are fortunate not to have had such problems occur whilst our patients have been exercising.

Coronary heart disease in any individual seems to be in a constant state of change, and disturbances in cardiac rhythm can arise in a patient who has never experienced them before. This serves to emphasize the extreme caution required when interpreting a stress test for the prescription of exercise. One of the advantages of having patients monitor their pulse rates and assess their reactions to exercise and everyday activities is that they thus become highly sensitized to a change in their own perception of health and will inform the physician if they are concerned. In many instances where genuine problems have developed, the early warnings have been extremely helpful.

It is important the patient should be aware of the need for adherence to a training regimen. Three 45-minute sessions per week is the ideal. Occasionally there is no harm whatsoever in missing one session per week, and this will have no effect at all on existing functional capacity. Training for only one session per week is not good enough and will have very little influence on cardiovascular fitness. The patient who decides to go for a once a month jog when the weather is fine is probably placing himself in danger and would be better not exercising at all. In this instance you are placing an unnecessary strain on an unfit system which is already damaged. If you decide not to exercise following your heart attack, then you must restrict your activities to your level of fitness. If you wish to acquire fitness, then there are no short cuts – you must be prepared to put in the effort and time if you are to experience the very beneficial dividends.

We have emphasized that a minimum of effort is required to attain a good standard of fitness. It is equally important to recognize that following a heart attack care and sensitivity are required throughout the training regimen. This is a classic example of where we can categorically state that *more* is not better. Target heart rates must be strictly adhered to while the injured system is healing and responding to graded work. Patience is certainly a virtue because time and common sense are critical features during the first year of rehabilitation.

There is much to be gained by exercising patients in groups because the social and psychological effects are extremely valuable. Inherent in this, however, are the problems of competition. Individuals tend to ignore their target heart rates and run with friends. Even in the least competitive situation friendly rivalry can sometimes develop. This is very unwise. The golden rule of all training principles is that the responses are individual. Training is always prescribed on an individual basis. With the post-coronary patient we are talking about a medical history that highlights the need for a personalized exercise programme. It is absolutely essential that the post-coronary patient recognizes this.

What then are the immediate benefits to be gained from exercise following a heart attack? The psychological and social benefits are easy to see but difficult to quantify. There is a very positive change in mood and emotion and this re-birth of self-confidence is an extremely important characteristic in the exercising patient. How much these emotional and mood changes are the result of the group interaction as opposed to changes coinciding with an improvement in functional capacity, is difficult to assess.

From the physiological point of view, our data and the data from similar studies show very clearly that trained post-coronary patients acheve physical performance levels equal to those of normal sedentary individuals. It would seem that training improves both the heart muscle and the circulation in addition to the skeletal muscle. The variability of response to training is much greater among coronary patients because of the range of extent of the myocardial damage. The influence of physical conditioning on the frequency and severity of recurring myocardial infarction (heart attack) has not been clearly defined using samples large enough to achieve statistical significance. However, results from recent studies using pooled data are much more encouraging and do suggest that there is a significnt reduction in recurrence rates among those individuals who are exercising as opposed to their non-exercising counterparts.

In conclusion, we strongly encourage the post-coronary patient, the angina patient and the post-bypass patient to become involved in a scientifically prescribed, medically monitored exercise programme. From our personal experience with many hundreds of patients we are convinced that the outstanding benefits far outweigh the small risk associated with the attainment of physical fitness.

9

Exercise – the Risks

One of the most common misconceptions among the lay public and medical profession alike is that fitness and health are synonymous. It is often assumed that if a person is healthy he must also be reasonably fit, and usually assumed that if he is obviously very fit, that he must of necessity be healthy. In fact the terms mean quite different things, and the distinction is an important one. Put simply, fitness can be regarded as the capacity to perform work, whilst health implies the absence of bodily disease. It follows that it is perfectly possible to be healthy but unfit (most individuals today would fall into this category), but equally possible to be very fit but unhealthy.

Sudden Death During Exercise

On Friday 20 July 1984, Jim Fixx, the man who was regarded by many as the father of the fitness movement in America and who provided the clarion call for many millions of Americans to take up 'jogging', collapsed and died on the Vermont State Highway. He was 52 years old and was out for his customary daily run when the tragedy occurred. At the post-mortem it was found that Jim Fixx had extensive underlying coronary heart disease, with two out of the three vessels supplying the heart extensively involved. There was also some evidence that he had actually sustained a number of small heart attacks in the past, and many people were frankly astonished that he could have continued with such a high level of physical activity, given the state of his coronary arteries.

Jim Fixx was an example of a man who was undoubtedly fit, but also very unhealthy. It is a strange irony that a man who, probably more than any other, had such an enormous impact on the activity patterns of so many Americans, should have fallen prey to the disease which is so clearly associated with sedentary lifestyles. The event was, of course, extensively reported in the media, apparently lending weight to the arguments of some that exercise is bad for you.

Of course Jim Fixx is only one example of many such tragedies that have occurred in recent years. Among the most famous was Vladimir Kutz, the Olympic 5,000 and 10,000 metre champion, who died in 1975 following a heart attack at the age of 48. In this section we shall consider in some detail the most serious potential risk during exercise, which is cardiac damage or sudden death. Whilst they are relatively uncommon occurrences, events such as the death of Jim Fixx tend to attract a disproportionate amount of coverage in the media, resulting in considerable concern and confusion among the population as a whole.

It must be said that most cases of sudden death that occur in Western countries have, of course, nothing to do with exercise. Tens of thousands of people die suddenly from cardiac disease each year, and the only relationship exercise has to these deaths is the fact that the victims did not take enough of it. When the press report the death of a well-known person, however, they have a tendency to distort the facts. It is often stated that the person concerned was very fit, that he ran or played squash regularly, and yet he died suddenly of a heart attack. A clear association is made between exercise and death. A closer inspection of the facts in most cases reveals that the person did not actually die *during* exercise. He was simply someone who took exercise on a reasonably regular basis and who happened to have a heart attack. The fact that he was known to take exercise is not directly relevant to his demise, except in so far as he may have died many years earlier if he had *not* been involved in physical activity.

Implicit in reporting of this kind is the idea that somehow exercise should have prevented the person's succumbing to heart disease. An association is often made between physical activity and immunity from heart disease without any evidence to support such an assumption. The death of Jim Fixx and others that are known to have occurred during or shortly after exercise raise important and disturbing questions. Did Fixx have any symptoms that may have warned him of his problem? Do most people who die during exercise have symptoms? Did running shorten or prolong Fixx's life, and did he run too much or not enough? In particular, why did not running or exercise in general protect him from heart disease? We will try to answer some of these questions.

Why Doesn't Exercise Provide Immunity from Heart Disease?

The fact that people die during exercise should not come as a surprise. Most males over the age of 40 in Western society, have some degree of narrowing of their coronary arteries, and a smaller number have a degree of involvement which is likely to place them at increased risk during vigorous exercise. If a heart is diseased it is common sense to suppose that the more vigorous the work required of it, the more likely it is to break down in some way. However, by far the vast majority of deaths due to heart disease are not directly associated with physical activity; they occur when people are driving their cars, working in their office or watching television.

The most important point to understand, however, is that physical activity is only one factor of importance in protection against heart disease. There are several other major factors, and we have already discussed the importance of cigarette smoking, high blood cholesterol, hypertension and family history. There is some reason to suppose that lack of exercise may be the most crucial factor, since increasing physical activity patterns tends to have a beneficial effect on the majority of the remaining risk factors. Nevertheless, the others cannot be ignored if the maximum protection is to be achieved.

If a person has a very high level of cholesterol in his bloodstream, it is imperative that he should make some effort to correct this, either by dietary means or through drugs if necessary. Running will not compensate for increased cholesterol levels. As an extreme example, if a person smokes 20 cigarettes per day, has a high blood cholesterol level because he eats the wrong diet, has a very strong family history of heart disease and has slightly elevated blood pressure, the fact that he may run 60 miles per week offers him no insurance. We must guard against giving the impression that exercise is the *only* factor to consider, when it is the *combination* of risk factors which is so important.

In Jim Fixx's case, there were several such factors evident in his history. First, he had previously been a heavy cigarette smoker and was also obese. He had turned to running as a means of improving his poor health and fitness. There was also some evidence that he had a personality Type A profile, and although we do not have any details concerning the levels of his blood cholesterol, it was known that he did not pay any particular attention to his diet in terms of his intake of animal fats. Finally, and this is a factor of great importance, Fixx's father died prematurely from heart disease at the age of 43, although it seems that his first heart attack was sustained when he was just 35. We must stress that anyone with a strong family history of coronary heart disease will not necessarily suffer premature disability or death themselves. It is simply that this is one other significant risk factor, and if you continue to smoke heavily and eat a poor diet, you are compounding your risk many times over.

There is some suggestion that Jim Fixx may have taken up running because he was frightened of suffering the same fate as his father. Had he paid a little more attention to other possible risk factors in his lifestyle, he may have been more successful. On a more positive note, however, it is quite possible that Jim Fixx would have died many years earlier had he not taken to running as a means of improving his health. Running may well have prolonged his life, and although one could never prove that this was the case, there is no doubt that exercise gave him a tremendous quality of life which it would be foolish to ignore.

We believe that exercise is able to exert its most powerful protective effects when it is started at a very early age and continued throughout life. Immunity to coronary artery disease has been reported in the Masai warriors who herd cattle on foot and the Tarahumara Indians who take part in ceremonial runs. For these groups high levels of physical activity are a way of life.

What Causes Death in Cases of Sudden Collapse during Physical Activity?

The vast majority of cases of sudden death during exercise are due to underlying coronary heart disease. The progressive blocking of the arteries supplying the heart which we explained in chapters 2 and 3 may progress to a point where insufficient blood is able to reach the heart during vigorous physical exertion. This may result in a blood clot forming at the site of the blockage, to cause a heart attack or 'coronary thrombosis', or it may result in a relative lack of oxygen to certain parts of the heart, causing the heart to become electrically unstable.

We have seen that the normal heart beats regularly, usually at a rate of 72 contractions per minute. In situations where the heart becomes short of oxygen, the heart may develop an abnormality in rhythm, which can prove fatal. The sequence in summary is as follows: an underlying blockage of coronary arteries (atheroma) leads to lack of blood to the heart muscle (ischaemia) or even to a fully formed blood clot totally stopping the flow of blood and therefore oxygen to a part of the heart muscle (thrombosis). Either of these factors may give rise to a sudden abnormality in cardiac rhythm and precipitate sudden death. When the heart goes into an abnormal rhythm it is unable to pump blood efficiently. This means that the blood and therefore the oxygen supply to the brain is impaired, and as a result loss of consciousness may ensue. Unless normal cardiac rhythm is restored within a few minutes, irreversible brain damage will occur.

Other disorders of the heart will occasionally be responsible for cardiac catastrophies during physical activity. Most cases of sudden death in young people, i.e. below the age of 35, are not actually due to coronary artery disease, but to a disease of the heart muscle itself (cardiomyopathy). This condition is sometimes hereditary, and is not caused by the same

Table 9.1   Causes of death during exercise in a sample of 109 deaths

Cause	Number
Coronary artery disease	80
Cardiomyopathy (heart muscle disease)	15
Congenital disease of coronary arteries	8
Inflammation of heart muscle	
(myocarditis)	3
Conduction defects	2
Ruptured aorta	1
Total	109

factors as those that are known to produce the progressive 'furring-up' of the blood vessels which is so typical of coronary artery disease. Apart from various kinds of heart muscle disease, there are occasions when congenital* abnormalities of the coronary arteries can cause problems during physical exertion. These are fortunately rare, but they do occasionally occur, particularly in the very young.

Finally, other causes of sudden death during exercise are spontaneous haemorrhage into the brain (sub-arachnoid haemorrhage) and inflammations of the heart muscle (myocarditis). These causes are infrequent, as will be seen from table 9.1.

Can the Risk be Quantified?

One of the problems about quantifying the relative risk in statistical terms is that the true incidence of sudden death during physical activity in this country is not known with any certainty. In addition, cases of sudden death *following* vigorous physical activity, for example 24 hours later, which may be due to damage to the heart muscle sustained during exercise, are extremely difficult to quantify. Many people dismiss the problem as being too small to merit special attention. We believe that while we can be fairly sure that the numbers are small, they are nevertheless greater than some would be prepared to admit. A number of deaths have been reported following marathons in this country, but this will not be the true number because such deaths are often under-reported, and the relationship of the death to physical exercise is often omitted from the death certificate. In addition, such cases are not adequately investigated, and some may not even be referred for post-mortem. The following case can serve as an example.

* A congenital abnormality is one which is present from birth, and which may or may not be hereditary.

We once performed tests in our laboratory on a 46-year-old man, including an exercise stress test. He was involved in regular physical activity of quite a vigorous kind, and was entirely free of symptoms. Because he felt so well he found it very difficult to accept the advice we offered. The results of his tests, and in particular his exercise test, indicated that he had extensive underlying heart disease. While accepting the limitations of this kind of investigation, the test was so unequivocally positive that we were bound to recommend he should undergo further tests, including coronary angiography. If he was not prepared to accept our offer of further tests, we felt very strongly that he should at least consider substantially reducing the intensity of his exercise programme. Neither of these two alternatives was apparently acceptable to him, and he continued to disregard the advice until his sudden death during vigorous exercise some 12 months later. Despite his sudden demise, no post-mortem was subsequently performed, and no mention made on his death certificate of the possible role of physical exertion in precipitating his premature death.

Workers in other countries have made some effort to quantify the number of cases of sudden death during various sporting activities. Using information from the Rhode Island Medical Examiner in the USA, Thomson and colleagues estimated that one death per 7,620 joggers occurred in the period from 1975 to 1980, equating to one death per 396,000 hours of jogging. In South Africa, Opie calculated the risk of sudden death among rugby players and referees. One sudden death occurred for every 50,000 rugby hours for the players, and for the referees it was one death for every 3,000 rugby hours. In Canada, Shepherd estimated one death per 2,500 gymnasium hours among middle-aged business men who attended unsupervised gymnasium programmes. This estimate, however, was based upon reports of such deaths reaching Ontario newspapers, and may therefore be an under-estimate. Of 2,606 sudden deaths in Finland, only 22 were associated with sports – 16 with skiing, two with jogging and four with other activities, an incidence of 0.8 per cent, compared to a 2.2 per cent incidence of sudden death among Finnish sauna bathers. It is surprising in view of this work done elsewhere that, despite a large number of exercise-associated deaths reported by the media in Britain, very few detailed studies of its incidence have been made.

To place the risk in perspective, one must bear in mind that approximately 1,000 sudden cardiac deaths occur daily in the USA. It is not known how many of these may have been precipitated by exercise, although the consensus of opinion is that exercise will increase the risk of sudden death in subjects with coronary heart disease. Nevertheless, there seems little doubt from the available evidence that the risk of dying during physical activity is generally very small, and also that the risk is not spread evenly throughout all groups. People with established risk factors for heart disease, who have been sedentary for long periods, may, as we shall see later, be especially vulnerable.

Is There Any Warning?

There is some suggestion that Jim Fixx, for example, may have had symptoms for some time prior to his death, but chose to ignore them. The element of denial is an important one, and may be related to a degree of addiction to exercise which those who are involved in exercise themselves will fully appreciate. While in most cases it is reasonable to term this a 'beneficial addiction', when it leads to denial of significant symptoms it may have serious consequences.

Many cardiologists believe Fixx must have experienced symptoms of some kind, given the extent of his underlying heart disease. However, there is much evidence to show that some individuals with gross coronary heart disease can and do perform high levels of physical exertion without any significant symptoms. We ourselves have seen a number of young individuals who have taken part in strenuous games of squash and other vigorous physical activity, without any symptoms at all, and yet on subsequent investigation were found to have extensive heart disease requiring, in some cases, corrective cardiac surgery.

From the facts available, however, it is likely that Fixx did have warning of problems for some time before his death. A few weeks before he had apparently told his son of a pain in his jaw and throat during exercise which he did not apparently regard as serious. He also complained of intermittent chest pain and of a particularly severe, prolonged episode of pain some four years previously.

One of the problems with the build-up of fatty plaque in the arteries is that in itself it is a painless process, and causes no symptoms. Only when the narrowing in the artery has progressed to the point where it begins to interfere with the blood supply to a particular organ do symptoms manifest themselves. In addition, there are some individuals who will suffer no symptoms at all, and in whom the first manifestation of a problem may be sudden death itself. In many cases, however, symptoms do become apparent but may not be recognized.

Classic pain from the heart is described as a crushing pain across the front of the chest, sometimes spreading into the arms and associated with pins and needles in the fingers. There may also be breathlessness or sweating. Clearly anyone exhibiting symptoms of this sort during exercise or at any other time should seek expert medical advice. However, the heart is a great deceiver, and occasionally unusual symptoms, which the individual may not immediately associate with heart problems, may be the first manifestation of the disease. Pain in the jaw, the teeth, or in the throat, may all be significant, but particularly so when they are consistently related to exertion. Sometimes there may only be pain in an arm or a shoulder (usually the left), and very often patients will not even describe the sensation as a pain but will complain of a *discomfort*, which they may not relate to cardiac problems.

In some cases the initial symptoms (prodromal symptoms), may be even more vague, making it more unlikely that the individual will make any association between his symptoms and cardiac problems. Sometimes there may be a vague feeling of nausea, breathlessness or a constant complaint of exhaustion, or just a sense of not feeling well. Fatigue, especially chronic fatigue, is sometimes an extremely important indicator of impending problems with the heart.

It may be difficult in some cases, therefore, to realize that the vaguer symptoms, very often the sort that most people would tend to brush off as being of no significance, may in reality be highly significant. Despite this, we need to bear in mind that not all cases of chest pain or pain in the jaw or teeth are necessarily due to heart disease. There are many other causes, including problems with the lower part of the oesophagus (gullet), which are not of any great significance. Clearly not everyone who has a feeling of tiredness or who feels vaguely unwell has heart problems. Common things occur commonly, and a person may feel unwell for many other reasons, for example lack of sleep or an underlying viral infection.

That said, however, if any of the following symptoms occur consistently in an individual, especially a middle-aged male, medical advice should be sought:

- Crushing chest pain related to exertion, which may spread into the arms or into the jaw, and which may be accompanied by pins and needles in the fingers (paraesthesia).
- Pain in the teeth, jaw or throat, consistently related to exertion.
- A burning sensation in the chest, throat or jaw, or sensation of tightness in these areas related to physical exertion.
- Dizziness, nausea, discomfort in the stomach, and inappropriate breathlessness related to exertion.
- Chronic fatigue, malaise and exhaustion.

Any of these symptoms, and any combination of these symptoms, particularly when related to exertion and occurring in a person with known risk factors for heart disease, should be discussed with a medical practitioner. Remember that if there is a definite relationship between the symptoms and physical activity, it is more likely to be significant.

Finally, on a more optimistic note, it should be remembered that most of us have odd 'twinges' from time to time, and these can occur in the upper body and chest as well as other places. These are most often due to minor strains and sprains in the ribs or in the muscles, and are usually associated with sharp pains, localized to one spot. This sort of pain, even when associated with physical exertion, is more often than not entirely innocent, and is not associated with cardiac problems.

The Addiction/'Immortality' Syndrome

Anyone involved in exercise prescription, or who works among people with high profiles of activity, will be well aware of the addictive properties of exercise. We have discussed the basis for this in chapter 5, but apart from any theoretical considerations, the phenomenon also has very considerable practical importance.

In our laboratory it is very common to observe certain groups of individuals who, to a greater or lesser degree, become addicted to their programmes of exercise. Some will no doubt object to the use of the term, but since we also believe that exercise can in many ways be regarded as a drug, it seems appropriate to describe the very real compulsion that certain people feel to perform exercise as an addiction. It is by no means uncommon to treat recurrent injuries in those who refuse to stop exercising and allow the damage to heal. They return time after time with breakdown following breakdown, and seem almost incapable of understanding that the prerequisite for full recovery is adequate rest. We have known some individuals with radiographically proved stress fractures who have continued to hobble around the streets, and we have also known marathon runners to compete with chest infections and all manner of other ailments. We would also suggest that anything that induces a normal individual to run ten miles in freezing temperatures or in pouring rain must have a compulsive or addictive element.

Most people who exercise with any regularity will admit that there is an element of addiction, however slight. In itself this is no bad thing, indeed we expect individuals for whom we prescribe exercise programmes to become addicted to some degree, which will serve as the spur for them to continue to benefit from their exercise. Most people recognize the compulsive quality of exercise and manage to keep it in perspective.

For others, however, their running programme, or whatever form of exercise they are involved in, becomes the most important thing in their lives. We have seen wives become 'exercise widows'. Indeed, exercise can become paramount to an absurd degree, with friends, marriage, children and occupation all assuming secondary importance. We have found this sort of addiction to be more common among runners than most other sporting groups and in particular among those who come to exercise late in

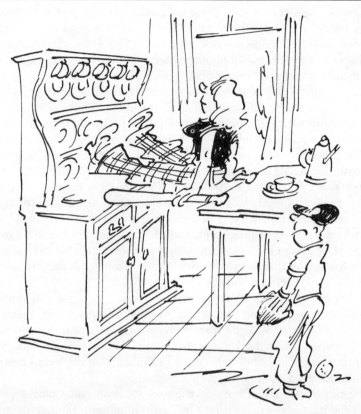

their lives. It is clear that training for a marathon requires a considerable commitment in terms of time. Running 100 miles per week or even more, and holding down a full-time job, does not leave a great deal of time for family, friends or other forms of more social recreation. It can become an obsession to the point where it becomes unhealthy. This is not meant to suggest that everyone should stop running marathons, but simply that they must accept the addictive quality of exercise and make sure that it does not result in very real hardship and stress for those around them.

We have discussed the question of immunity from coronary heart disease, and shown that exercise in itself does not provide full insurance cover against heart attack or even sudden death. There is no doubt that if you exercise you are far less likely to suffer the consequences of heart disease, but that is not the same as being immune.

The issue of immunity dates to a large extent from a statement by a Californian pathologist, Thomas Bassler. He claimed that anyone who could complete a marathon inside four and a half hours and who was also a non-smoker, would be immune from coronary heart disease for the next five years. This contentious point aroused great controversy, although many people were apparently convinced. His claim received wide press coverage, mainly because it was so controversial, but the press did not give similar coverage to the data published later that showed very clearly that the 'Bassler imperative' was wrong.

Many reports have now appeared in the literature documenting coronary heart disease in athletes, including marathon runners. Noakes and Opie in South Africa helped to destroy the 'immunity' myth by documenting sudden deaths from heart disease in several marathon runners. Their data included one 44-year-old man who had completed eight marathons and two ultramarathons in the 14 months prior to his sudden death at the 19 km point of a 24 km road race. Post-mortem revealed extensive coronary artery disease, with evidence of an acute myocardial infarction (heart attack). This man was a non-smoker, but he did have a high blood cholesterol level, confirming that exercise did not provide immunity in the setting of other significant risk factors. Again, exercise may have allowed him to live longer than he would otherwise have done, but there is no clear evidence to support such a claim.

Waller also describes many cases of severe heart disease and death in conditioned runners over the age of 40, two of whom were marathon runners. All five of Waller's cases were proved to have extensive three-vessel coronary artery disease at post-mortem. It is interesting to note once again that both the marathon runners in Waller's sample were known to have raised blood cholesterol levels.

These cases are important because they illustrate some crucial points about the irrational yet persistent belief in 'immunity' through exercise. When the exercise addiction is combined with a belief in immunity from heart disease via exercise, the combination can be lethal. The unfounded sense of 'immortality' which many such individuals feel may encourage them to deny significant symptoms during exercise that may be an early warning of serious problems. The kind of deception that occurs probably runs something like this: 'This pain which I am having at present cannot be pain from my heart. I couldn't run the way I do and have heart disease. Running all these miles must have given me a strong and healthy heart, maybe if I push a little harder the pain will go away.' In the words of the ultramarathoner Dennis Coffee, 'You gotta be brave to be a runner. We're all tough guys.'

Many people still believe this kind of mythology, and when they eventually visit their own general practitioner, he may even tend to agree with them. Many doctors would still believe that anyone who is a marathon runner would be extremely unlikely to have heart disease. Depending upon other factors, he is certainly *less likely* to have underlying problems, but each problem requires very careful assessment. We have had considerable experience with the 'addiction/immortality' syndrome. In some unfortunate individuals the result was catastrophic. In others it has had less serious consequences, and they were able to continue exercising at a lower intensity.

One last case history will illustrate the points we have been seeking to make.

OL was 48 years old and a regular runner who attended our department for evaluation of his fitness and his cardiac state. He had a history of symptoms that was suggestive although not diagnostic of heart disease, and he had expressed an interest in running marathons. Although his exercise electrocardiograph was essentially normal, we were not happy with the situation and recommended that he should reduce the intensity of his exercise, and report any further deterioration in his symptoms. He later returned to the laboratory, and reported that he had completed more than 2,000 miles in training, and had also competed in several half-marathons quite successfully. When questioned about symptoms, he admitted to occasional vague chest discomfort, but said this tended to disappear after only a few miles' running. His main request on this occasion was that we should predict his best marathon time from a further exercise test, since he intended entering a full marathon in the near future. Repeat evaluation in this man showed he was substantially fitter than previously, with a $\dot{V}O_2$ max of 53 ml kg^{-1} min^{-1}. The electrocardiograph during the test, however, was grossly abnormal, suggesting serious underlying coronary heart disease. He admitted to only vague pain during the test, although our impression was that there was some element of denial at work. Subsequent investigation, including coronary angiography, revealed extensive three-vessel disease which was not amenable to surgical correction.

This case illustrates the poor relationship between the extent of the disease and the symptoms, and the element of denial that was almost certainly present. In addition, this man also had a significantly raised cholesterol level, and in this respect is very similar to those cases documented by Noakes, mentioned previously. Finally it also illustrates the remorseless progression of heart disease in an individual with high levels of physical activity and fitness. This man is in fact continuing to run regularly, but has agreed to modify substantially the intensity of his exercise programme.

Can Those at Risk of Heart Attack or Death Be Identified?

We have seen that certain individuals involved in vigorous exercise may be at undue risk of suffering a cardiac catastrophe. The risk is very small, and very much less than the risk of avoiding exercise altogether. However, it would be greatly to our advantage if high risk individuals could be identified *prior* to becoming involved in exercise, in order that a programme could be prescribed individually and at an intensity that would be as safe as possible. Anything that can be done to reduce the small numbers of deaths during exercise deserves our attention.

First, those individuals at most risk are those with conventional coronary risk factors. Thus age, sex, blood pressure, family history of heart disease, blood cholesterol, cigarette smoking and stress all contribute to an increased risk, and the more risk factors an individual has, the greater the likelihood that he will succumb to heart disease. Many surveys of sudden death in exercise show that in the majority of cases the victims have one or more conventional coronary risk factors. In studies of squash players in this country, Northcote and Ballantyne found one or more of these risk factors in 73 per cent of those who had died during exercise. These data are confirmed in many other studies, and in our own work we found that those individuals who might be at risk during vigorous physical activity had one or more conventional risk factors in the majority of cases (80 per cent).

Exercise stress testing is also of use in identifying individuals at risk. Highly sophisticated systems are now available, incorporating computerized interpretation of the records. In our view, however, there is still no real substitute for the trained physician supervising the test, and analysing the data produced. A typical test in progress is illustrated in plate 3.

The reader must bear in mind that a resting electrocardiograph can give only very limited information about the condition of the heart. By making a recording while the heart is under an exercise load, as in an exercise stress test, a great deal more information can be obtained, making such testing a powerful diagnostic tool. Some doctors dispute the accuracy of exercise testing as a means of diagnosing coronary heart disease, and certainly the technique is not foolproof. However, in skilled and experienced hands, using the strictest criteria for interpretation, and when the technique is applied to populations where coronary heart disease is common, the test without question has a very high predictive value.

During a 12 month period we studied a large sample (1,000) of males in the age range 20–65 who were apparently healthy. Exercise testing was performed in all cases and only those who had no symptoms prior to the testing were included in the study. All had expressed an interest in improving their standard of fitness through a programme of progessive exercise. In summary, we identified a total of 80 patients (8 per cent) who, on the basis of electrocardiographic abnormalities during exercise testing, could be regarded as being at increased risk during vigorous physical activity. Several of these individuals were referred for more invasive investigations, and several subsequently underwent successful coronary bypass surgery. The important point to note is that these individuals were *apparently* healthy and that most of the positive tests results were found in individuals who had at least one or more conventional coronary risk factors.

Exercise stress testing is not widely available in this country, although it is now extensively employed in the USA. In our view, the ideal situation would be for all subjects who wanted to take part in exercise programmes, who were aged 35 years or more, to undergo an exercise stress test. We accept the practical limitations of such a policy, but feel that the investigation should be used in situations where, because of the presence of several coronary risk factors, the subject would be regarded as being in the 'high risk' category. Exercise programmes could then be prescribed for these individuals on the basis of individual physiological data.

Conclusions

The risk of sustaining a sudden cardiac catastrophe during exercise is small. Nevertheless, it is significant, and should not be ignored. The evidence would strongly suggest that there is a sub-group of individuals, most often first-time exercisers over the age of 40, with one or more conventional coronary risk factors, who may be at undue risk during vigorous physical activity. We believe that some of these subjects can be identified prior to becoming involved in exercise.

In chapter 6 we outlined a detailed screening procedure that can be applied relatively easily. We believe that those individuals who, after the initial assessment and the general practitioner assessment, are categorized in a high risk group should be referred for more detailed investigation, including exercise stress testing.

We have discussed the question of the risks involved in exercise in some detail because, as a result of increasingly frequent reports of exercise-related deaths which have paralleled the increase in leisure-time activity in recent years, many members of the public will be concerned and confused about the real risks involved. Although exercise-related deaths are becoming more frequent the phenomenon itself is not entirely new. After running to Athens from Marathon in 490 BC, bringing the news of victory over the Persians, Pheidippides, who was apparently a trained runner, is said to have collapsed and died! Nevertheless, we make the point again, that by far the greatest risk is *not* to exercise, and we would be fully in support of any programme or policy that encouraged what is still essentially a sedentary population in this country to become more active. We do believe, however, that the public is entitled to the facts and should know that exercise of moderate intensity, performed on a regular basis, has substantial benefits, but also carries a small but significant risk.

It is human nature to want to believe that a thing is all good or all bad. However, few things in life are that simple, and exercise is no exception. We believe that the simple screening system we have suggested would go at least some way towards identifying the high-risk individuals. We also believe that the public should be made more aware of possible symptoms during exercise, which may indicate underlying cardiac problems. Screening, together with increased vigilance and a more realistic view of the benefits of exercise, will help to reduce the number of exercise-induced cardiac catastrophes.

10

Exercise – Your Questions Answered

In recent years, the exercise 'movement' in this country and in the USA has been a particularly fertile breeding ground for health and fitness 'experts'. Some of these people have had a measurable degree of success as athletes themselves, but a greater number have no claim to any form of specialized knowledge. There is an assumption that those who have attractive bodies or have achieved a certain athletic prowess, are qualified to write about health. The logic is unsound. It is like assuming that the man who comes to read your electricity meter is an expert on nuclear fission.

The increasing interest in diet, exercise and health in general is, to a large extent, a product of the growing exercise 'industry' in this country. The growing interest in aerobics, dance classes, squash and marathon running has helped to create an atmosphere in which people are beginning to assume a greater responsibility for their own health. To this extent, the present exercise movement has made an important and real contribution to the health prospects of the population in general. Unfortunately, it has also attracted its fair share of self-styled 'experts' and fanatics. Much of the information currently available to the lay public concerning the benefits of exercise, diet and other health issues is misguided, sometimes banal and sometimes frankly dangerous. Most of it, however, is well intended. One of the major problems at present is that there is no clearly defined qualification for exercise and dance instructors, and so the quality of the teaching and advice given is disturbingly inconsistent. There is an urgent need for a recognizable 'professional' qualification and minimum standard for exercise teachers and it is time a professional institution or body was formed in order to bring such a qualification into being. In our judgement this would have a number of important benefits.

First, it would encourage greater numbers of the general public to

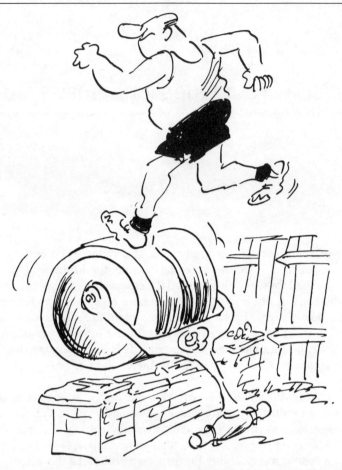

become involved in regular exercise programmes, including specialized programmes for the elderly. Exercise has been shown to be of great benefit in the elderly but, clearly, it needs to be applied with sensitivity and with skill if injuries and other problems are to be avoided. A group of professionally qualified exercise teachers would be able to apply properly supervised programmes of exercise to all sections of the community and all age groups.

Secondly, it would encourage a much higher quality of written material and this would mean, in turn, that much of the present mountain of literature on the subject could be consigned to where it truly belongs – the wastepaper bin.

Finally, a professional association of this kind would encourage doctors and other paramedical personnel to refer patients for specialized instruction and advice concerning the benefits of exercise. As a group, doctors, know very little about exercise, and it is unrealistic to expect them to do so. Many doctors would clearly welcome a professional organization of this kind, in which they would feel able to place their trust.

For a few people exercise has become a 'cause' to be pursued with an almost religious fervour. Like most minorities, such people are extremely vociferous, and their attitude and fervour, together with their completely unrealistic claims about the benefits of exercise, have turned many ordinary people against the idea of exercise forever. It is interesting that these people talk about fitness and health as though they were clearly understandable terms, and yet they themselves have probably thought very little about what these terms imply. Likewise 'health and fitness' magazines and journals abound and implicit in them is the assumption that everyone understands what the terms mean. We shall be giving some consideration to their definition, which is complex, at a later stage in this chapter.

In an atmosphere in which the pro-exercise movement has seemingly had full rein for some years, it was almost inevitable that an opposite reaction should occur. To some extent the very absurdities of the pro-exercise movement have made its devotees vulnerable to attack. The cynics have always been around, but in his book 'The Exercise Myth' (1985), Dr Henry Solomons mounted a scathing attack on the exercise movement, both in terms of its over-commercialization and also the scientific evidence on which it is based. Dr Solomons' book was not only inevitable, it was very welcome. It helped to restore a sense of perspective and reality to a twentieth century phenomena that some people felt was getting out of hand.

Unfortunately, the evidence Solomons presented in support of his argument was highly selective, and could not in any sense be regarded as a fair representation of the enormous amount of evidence that now exists supporting the exercise hypothesis. To this extent, the book has not been taken seriously, and it is sad that a member of the medical profession itself, which should be leading the cause, should have presented such a cynical and biased argument. Solomons also ignored the 'spin-off' effects of exercise, e.g. giving up smoking or changing one's diet, and these effects are of the greatest importance.

The exercise movement in the USA has encouraged thousands of Americans to adopt a more responsible attitude towards their own health and this must account, in no small part, for the major reductions in coronary disease that have been observed in that country during the past 15–20 years. In this sense, and this is by far the most important, the exercise movement has been of immeasurable benefit.

Attitudes in Britain are also beginning to change, and many people are now asking searching questions about the attitude of the medical profession, which thus far has failed to provide any major impetus towards prevention. Many doctors recognize the need for fundamental changes and are enthusiastic and well-informed with regard to measures of prevention. Unfortunately, many others are slow to change and remain cynical, clinging to old, established ideas.

The pro-exercise fanatics will imply that exercise is the panacea for all ills, and will prevent or cure almost anything. The anti-exercise movement, of which Dr Solomons is a representative, claims that exercise has absolutely no proved benefit whatsoever. As always, the truth lies somewhere between the two extremes. The evidence that exercise has a major contribution to play in combating disease is compelling. However, it is but one factor among many others and it is a more complete and balanced overall approach which is required.

In our everyday practice we have to advise an enormous number of people on a wide range of health issues, including exercise. Our patients will include those with severe cardiac disease, children with spina bifida, paraplegics, overweight businessmen, weekend joggers and, at the other end of the spectrum, world-class and Olympic athletes. Despite the variation in ability, we find that certain questions tend to recur again and again. The following is a cross-section of the most common questions, and each is followed by a comment or a short explanatory paragraph. Much of the information in the answers will be found elsewhere in the book. Nevertheless, we felt it would be useful to bring together some concise information with regard to specific questions in a way that we hope will be more accessible.

Questions and Answers

What Exactly is Health or Being Healthy?

Most of us feel instinctively that we know exactly what being healthy means. Actually, the term is not amenable to precise definition, and a few moments' reflection will alow us to appreciate that it is, in fact, quite a complex concept. When we talk about disease, we are talking about an essentially negative concept. Lack of ease, or dis-ease, implies a state in which the psychological and physical harmony and equilibrium of the body are in some way threatened. This may be due to easily definable causes, such as cancer, or a simple cold, and we are conventionally quite content to refer to both these conditions as diseases. However, disease can arise from a variety of sources and the threat to the organism may not be so easily quantifiable or recognizable.

For example, certain life events, such as divorce or bereavement, certainly cause a sense of disharmony, but most of us would not refer to the psychological state which ensues from these events as being a diseased state. But in the broadest sense in which we have used the term, i.e., lack of ease or dis-ease, then distress following divorce, bereavement or similar events certainly does qualify as a disease. It is simply that we conventionally refer to disease states as conditions in which we can see a clearly definable and quantifiable cause, usually physical in orgin. When we move on to psychological difficulties, we are much less amenable to using the term disease. Being a heroin addict or alcoholic undoubtedly leads to disease, but would we be prepared to accept these conditions as diseases in the conventional sense?

When we turn to the question of being healthy, or being in a state of good health, we are not simply implying the absence of disease. Being healthy is much more than this. In the same way that lack of ease is a negative concept, then being healthy is a positive concept. It is a sense of 'wellness', which again is not amenable to precise definition. It encompasses a number of feelings, such as exhilaration at the sheer joy of being alive, a sense of wellness and harmony and a sense of being at peace with both ourselves and others. It implies a state of wellness not only physically but also psychologically, and the existence of a clear state of harmony between both the psychological and physical aspects of our make-up. Lack of disease is not the same as being healthy. Each of us needs a sense of fulfilment and a sense of progress and worth in our lives to feel fully alive and healthy.

What Exactly is Fitness?

In strict physiological terms fitness can be defined as the capacity to perform work. However, a few moments reflection quickly reveal the inadequacy of such a definition. First, when most people think about fitness they tend to think about some form of sporting activity, for example, badminton, squash, cycling, running etc. Yet even those among us who exercise regularly will only spend a very tiny fraction of their lives performing such physical activity. Apart from running, cycling etc. we perform many hundreds of other forms of physical activity every day, from washing the dishes to walking the dog. Any definition of fitness, therefore, will have to take into account such variations in physical activity.

Secondly, we have to consider what kind of fitness we are talking about. The physical demands of running a seven-minute mile are not the same as pushing a heavy wheelbarrow all day or pushing a pen in a sedentary occupation. Thus the physical demands or requirements vary enormously from individual to individual and any concept of fitness must take such variations into account.

Thirdly, is there not a psychological component to be considered? Any definition of fitness, if it is to be adequate, must also take into account our mental state.

Finally, we also know there is a minimum level of physical exercise required to maintain and promote health, and this must also be included.

Given these considerations, a possible definition of fitness, or more properly of a 'readiness for living' can be stated as follows: Fitness, or 'readiness for living' can be defined as *the ability of the individual to cope with the mental and physical demands of living and to perform sufficient physical exercise to promote and maintain health.*

What is the Relationship Between Fitness and Health?

The true answer to this question is that there is not necessarily any relationship at all. It is perfectly possible to be healthy and yet unfit. It is equally possible, although less likely, to be fit and yet not healthy. We have a number of patients who have quite a high degree of cardiovascular fitness but who, on subsequent investigation, turned out to have severe or even life-threatening disease. Feeling well is absolutely no guarantee of good health: most people who have heart attacks feel well the day before. However, from a practical point of view, a trained person who is highly physically active is much less *likely* to be unhealthy.

If Cigarette Smoking and these So-called 'Risk Factors' Are So Bad for You, Why Did Uncle Albert, Who Smoked 40 Full-strength Cigarettes a Day, Ate Dripping Sandwiches and Never Did a Scrap of Exercise Live to be 93?

This is a common question and one which many people find difficult to understand. There is no cause and effect relationship between the risk factors we have described and the development of disease. If you are a heavy cigarette smoker, it does not necessarily follow that you will develop lung cancer or heart disease; the converse of that statement, however, is that lung cancer in non-smokers is a relatively rare condition. In other words, as far as lung cancer is concerned, cigarette smoking is a necessary but not sufficient prerequisite to the development of the disease. All one can say is that if you smoke 40 cigarettes a day, then your risk of developing lung cancer or heart disease is very substantially greater than if you did not smoke.

In the same way, eating large amounts of fat in your diet does not make it certain you will develop heart disease, it simply means that the *risk* of your so doing is substantially greater. In addition, you must also remember that the risk factors work with each other to increase the risk even further. For example, cigarette smoking in combination with high blood pressure will more than double the risk and the addition of high blood cholesterol to these two factors will increase the risk by a factor of eight. In a study of British physicians it was shown that 40 per cent of 35-year-old men who smoked more than 25 cigarettes per day, died before the age of 65, compared with 15 per cent of non-smokers in the same category. In addition, the risk of developing lung cancer is quantitatively related to cigarette smoke exposure. Men who smoke one packet of cigarettes a day increase their risk tenfold compared with non-smokers; men who smoke two packets a day increase their risk more than 25-fold. Cigarette smoking is also powerfully associated with coronary heart disease and with a number of other serious conditions.

There is only one way to play Russian Roulette safely, and that is with an empty gun. However, there will always be some people (and this presumably includes Uncle Albert) who will play the game with five bullets in the gun and still get away with it. Most, however, do not.

Is it Better to Smoke a Pipe or Cigars rather than Cigarettes?

Overall the death rates of pipe smokers and cigar smokers are very substantially lower than those of cigarette smokers. It is not known exactly why pipe and cigar smoking should be relatively safer but it is probably due in part to such factors as differences in smoke constituents, temperature, degree of acidity or alkalinity and the tendency for cigar and pipe smokers to inhale much less than cigarette smokers. If you must smoke, therefore, a pipe or an occasional cigar is a very much safer alternative to cigarettes. You should bear in mind, however, that cancer rates for the mouth, larynx and the digestive tract are the same in cigar, pipe and cigarette smokers.

Is Involuntary Smoking or 'Passive' Smoking Significant?

There is absolutely no doubt that passive or involuntary smoke inhalation can have an adverse effect upon health. One cannot always choose to be in a smoke-free environment, but smoke can be extremely irritating to the eyes and has a definite deleterious effect on those with angina and chronic lung disease. In addition, a number of studies have shown that the risk of cancer is more than doubled for the spouse of a smoker who smokes less than one packet a day and more than tripled for those whose spouses smoke more than one packet a day. Cancer of the lung is an unfortunate tragedy at any time, but to develop this condition from *someone else's* cigarette smoking is a scandal.

Other forms of passive smoking are also important. It is now well recognized that babies of mothers who smoke tend to be lighter at birth and that pregnant mothers who smoke increase their chance of miscarriage. There is also some evidence that the long-term development of the child may be hindered.

There are also studies that show that the children of parents who smoke suffer frequently from respiratory disease such as bronchitis because in a child's smaller body and smaller lungs, the effects are greater.

So, in summary, if possible do not smoke at all, *ever*; if you must smoke, stick to a pipe or cigars and whatever you smoke KEEP IT TO YOUR-SELF.

Is Reducing Salt Intake Really Helpful?

A number of committees examining the relationship between diet and health, including the Committee on Medical Aspects of Food Policy, have recommended a substantial reduction in the national intake of salt. This is because there is thought to be an association between high salt intake and the development of hypertension (high blood pressure). Whilst there is by no means complete agreement among the various experts, there does, however, seem to be a consensus emerging that high salt diets may be a major factor in precipitating high blood pressure in a certain section of the population. It is not known by what mechanism this occurs, although it may be due to genetic differences in the ability of the kidney to handle high salt loads.

It is not possible at the present time to identify those individuals in the population who are 'salt-sensitive'. It is not easy, either, to place a figure on what sort of percentage may be at risk. There is no question that in the clinical setting of treating patients with hypertension many are able to achieve quite dramatic reductions in their resting blood pressure by reducing their dietary salt intake. Certainly all patients with hypertension should endeavour to do this so far as possible. Since, in the population at large, we cannot identify the 'salt-sensitive' individuals, it would seem reasonable to advise a general reduction in salt intake for the population as a whole. There is no evidence that this recommendation would have any adverse effect on the health of the population and there is substantial evidence that a section of the population, albeit a minority, would benefit from such a reduction.

If you are trying to reduce the salt intake in your own diet, you should bear in mind that various forms of salt, such as sea salt, have no advantage at all over ordinary table salt. If you find that reducing your salt intake is too unpalatable, it may be worthwhile trying a salt substitute, such as potassium chloride. These are available under various names in most chemists, although not everyone finds them palatable.

Will Exercise Help Me to Live Longer?

A large part of this book has been discussing the question of the relationship between exercise and disease, in particular cardiovascular disease. If we accept that exercise helps to protect against heart disease, then clearly the probability that one will survive the allotted span, substantially increases. In the sense in which exercise will help to mitigate against the effects of adverse lifestyles, it may help indirectly to prolong life. Most studies have shown that exercise is actually an independent risk factor which exerts a beneficial effect irrespective of other risk factors such as high blood pressure and high blood cholesterol. However, if you were to take a perfect environment, in which diet, lifestyle etc. were precisely controlled for the benefit of the organism, it is not known precisely what effect regular exercise would have upon the ageing processes in the body. At the present time there is no evidence that, given that ideal environment, exercise would actually prolong cellular life.

The processes of ageing are highly complex and we have a great deal to learn about the changes in cellular structure which occur as a result of the ageing process. The authors would certainly not claim that exercise can exert any measurable benefit in this respect, simply because there is no available evidence. However, in the sense that physical exercise helps to promote health and well-being, then it can help us to be 'old' for a shorter period of time. Although you may not live any longer than three score years and ten, physical activity will help you to be active for a larger percentage of that allotted time. Some of our subjects in their sixties and seventies are, in physiological terms, ten or 20 years younger. Unfortunately, the converse is also true; we also see 30- and 40-year-old subjects who are physiologically 20 years older than their chronological age. We encourage individuals to be active for as long as possible, if only because we are absolutely sure this substantially improves their quality of life whilst not *necessarily* prolonging it beyond the expected lifespan.

Is the Resting Pulse Rate and the Ability of the Pulse to 'Recover' following Exercise, a Good Indicator of Cardiovascular Fitness?

The development of a slow resting heart rate, or a 'sinus bradycardia' to give it its correct medical name, is a normal effect of sustained endurance exercise. It is due to a number of factors, including an increase in tone in the vagus nerve which tends to slow the heart. In general, athletes have much slower heart rates than untrained individuals. The normal resting heart rate is approximately 70 beats per minute but it is not uncommon to find athletes with heart rates in the 40s or even lower. This denotes a large, powerful heart, which is able to accomplish its task in fewer contractions than the so-called normal heart. There are, however, a large number of other causes for a slow resting heart rate and so the mere fact of finding a slow pulse rate does not necessarily denote a state of health. As a rough guide, however, and in the setting of a history of regular, vigorous physical activity, it is a normal finding and suggests a degree of cardiovascular fitness above the average. It gives no indication as to the level of that fitness in terms of maximum oxygen consumption ($\dot{V}O_2$ max).

The rate of recovery of the pulse, that is the rate at which it returns to normal following vigorous exercise, is a rough guide to cardiovascular fitness. However, recovery rates vary enormously, even among highly trained individuals, and so it cannot be used as a means of predicting maximum aerobic capacity or the athletic ability of the individual concerned.

What is the Value of Exercise Stress Testing?

The use of exercise stress testing has attracted a certain amount of dissent and even controversy. Very often it is not the exercise test itself which is at fault, but the competence of the individuals who use it.

Any investigation in medicine has certain limitations. A chest X-ray can provide a certain amount of information but its accuracy depends on a multitude of factors, ranging from the technical quality of the film, to the experience and ability of the physician who is to interpret it. The important thing is to recognize the limitations of the investigation and to make the necessary allowances.

Exercise stress testing, like any other diagnostic tool, has limitations. However, in competent, skilful and experienced hands, it is a powerful and practical way of identifying cardiac disease. A strongly positive exercise test is powerful evidence in favour of underlying cardiac disease. We have seen a significant number of apparently healthy individuals who have undergone extensive cardiac surgery as a result of their heart condition being identified by an exercise stress test. It is true that a negative test does not provide any absolute guarantee that an individual is free of cardiac disease, but no test currently available will tell you that you will not have a heart attack. All we would say is that a negative exercise test is powerfully reassuring, and strongly indicates against the presence of life-threatening underlying disease.

In the next few years it is likely that exercise stress testing will be refined even further, and in conjunction with certain newly developed biochemical techniques, it will prove to be an even more powerful means of screening populations.

Will Exercise Prevent My Getting Heart Disease?

This question has been considered in detail in chapter 9, but it is worthwhile re-stating that regular, vigorous exercise will help to protect against coronary heart disease but it does *not* provide immunity. Exercise is but one factor amongst many and it is no more or less important than cigarette smoking or a high blood fat level.

Is Running 100 miles a Week better than Running 20 miles a Week?

The answer to this question revolves around the word 'better'. If you run a 100 miles a week then it is likely you will run a marathon faster than if you only run 20 miles a week. In terms of running marathons, therefore, 100 miles a week is better than running 20 miles a week. However, in terms of basic health and certainly in terms of any cardio-protective effect that exercise may have, there is not a scrap of evidence to suggest that running 100 miles a week is any more beneficial than running 20 miles a week. You may certainly be fitter, but it is unlikely that you will be any less prone to have a heart attack than someone of your own age and sex who is running 20 miles a week. The requirements of exercise in terms of basic cardiovascular fitness and the health benefits which this provides are fairly clear. Three or four 30-minute sessions of exercise a week is the requirement, and translated into running terms this means between 14 and 20 miles a week. If you run more than this your cardiovascular fitness will improve but you will not acquire any further protection against heart disease. In addition, in our experience, mileages much above 30 or 40 a week are accompanied by a substantial increase in bone, joint, tendon and muscle injuries.

Is it a Good Idea to Continue Exercising with a Cold in the Hope that the Exercise will 'Sweat it Out'?

There is still the idea amongst even experienced athletes that running with a head cold will help to 'sweat it out' and somehow facilitate a faster recovery. Nothing could be further from the truth. Indeed, we now know that it is postively dangerous to run with a cold or indeed any other infection. The reason is that the virus which causes a cold or influenza may, under certain circumstances, have a propensity to invade the heart muscle itself, a condition known as myocarditis. Myocarditis can be a serious disease, and while it is true that the chances of actually developing it are small, the possible consequences can be very serious indeed. The advice, therefore, must be that if you have a cold or other infection or illness, you positively should not exercise. Exactly how long you should wait before commencing exercise again varies between individuals. It is much better to wait until all the cold symptoms have disappeared entirely and then to start exercising again very gradually. Provided that you are careful and sensible, within a few days you will be exercising at your normal intensity and frequency.

It is important to recognize, however, that many subjects continue to feel unwell and complain of tiredness, malaise and lethargy for many weeks and even months after an illness. We do not yet know why such effects can continue for so long but we do know that resuming regular physical activities before the body has fully recovered can sometimes precipitate a relapse or a prolongation of symptoms. One of the most common problems in our own laboratory is helping athletes to recover from viral illnesses and get back to their original form. For many of them this is a long and difficult process, and in some instances full recovery is never achieved. Prospects of recovery are certainly not helped by impatience, nor by driving oneself hard physically before being capable of performing such exercise. It demands great patience and encouragement to bring such individuals back to full form and it is a salutary reminder of the sometimes profound effects on physical performance that viral infections can have. In addition, depression following viral infections of any kind is an extremely common phenomenon and again may take many weeks or months to subside.

In summary, therefore we should treat viral infections with great respect and our own policy is to advise people to lie low and be as physically inactive as possible during the course of the illness. When the symptoms have subsided it is reasonable gradually to resume your programme of normal activity, but at the same time you must be extremely sensitive to feelings of tiredness which may occur much earlier than usual. A simple piece of advice is, if you feel tired and uncomfortable, walk for a while or stop altogether and go home. We would emphasize that the vast majority of people make full and uncomplicated recoveries following such infections, but it is unwise for anyone to take unnecessary risks.

Will Exercise Help to Protect against Cancer?

There is, as yet, no firmly established relationship between physical activity patterns and cancer. This is hardly surprising since the association has never been studied in detail and cancer is not one disease but a whole range of highly complex disease states, which probably have a multiplicity of causes.

One recent study in the *American Journal of Epidemiology* reported an increased risk of bowel cancer in those individuals engaged in sedentary occupations. High activity jobs (jobs in which workers spend less than 20 per cent of their time sitting) posed the lowest risk. Those in moderately active jobs were 1.3 times more likely to develop cancer of the colon whilst those in sedentary jobs had a risk which was approximately 1.6 times that of the high activity workers. One obviously needs to be cautious about drawing too many firm conclusions from a study of this kind since there are clearly a wide range of other factors that need to be taken into account. Nevertheless, these initial results are encouraging and further research in this area will continue.

Both My Parents Suffered with Coronary Heart Disease. Does this Mean I Will Suffer the Same Problems?

The short answer is 'No', although there is clearly a somewhat increased risk of developing coronary disease yourself. It is not always easy to gauge the extent of genetic risk in any one individual, because any apparent genetic component may in fact be mediated by other inherited conditions. For example, if high blood pressure or high blood fats run in the family, then you have an increased risk of developing such conditions yourself and these are obviously major risk factors for the development of heart disease. It is also clear, however, that the genetic factor can act independently of these other conventional factors, and one may often find coronary heart disease running in families who have no obvious conventional coronary risk factors. This is very unusual, however, and more often than not there is a history of high blood pressure, high blood fats, cigarette smoking, obesity etc., which are obviously important in the development of coronary heart disease.

A family history of coronary heart disease, rather like age and male sex, is one of the conventional risk factors about which you can do nothing. However, it should serve as a warning and encourage you to concentrate on other possible risk factors that may be present, factors which may be amenable to manipulation. Thus, having your blood pressure and your blood fats measured at regular intervals, taking an interest in your diet and engaging in moderate physical activity would certainly be prudent.

In summary, a strong family history of coronary disease is a definite risk factor, but you should not worry about this unduly and should simply concentrate on making sure that whatever coronary risk factors are potentially under your control are dealt with accordingly.

How Much Exercise Should I Take?

This topic was dealt with in detail in chapter 7. In summary, we recommend three or four 20–30-minute sessions of exercise each week with the heart rate maintained during that period at approximately 75 per cent of

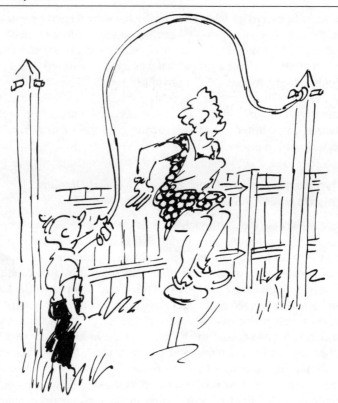

the heart rate reserve. The heart rate reserve is the difference between the resting heart rate and the age predicted maximum heart rate (APMHR). To calculate the APMHR subtract your age from 220. For example if you are 40, your APMHR is 180. The heart rate reserve is the APMHR minus the resting heart rate, so that if your resting heart rate is 70 then the heart rate reserve is $180 - 70 = 110$. We then take 75 per cent of 110, which equals 82 beats per minute. Finally we add the resting heart rate once again, which equals $82 + 70 = 152$. The correct intensity of exercise in this instance therefore is that which produces a heart rate of approximately 152 beats per minute. We have shown you how to count your pulse over a ten-second period in chapter 7.

We recommend a day of rest between each exercise session, although some people would prefer to exercise every day. This is not necessary to maintain cardiovascular fitness and there is evidence that fitness can actually be maintained on twice a week activity. In order to maintain and improve fitness, however, we recommend three or four sessions a week. Remember that the heart does not discriminate between types of exercise and so the exact type of physical exercise engaged in is not as important as the fact that it should involve major muscle groups, be regular and rhythmical .

If My Coronary Arteries Are Already Blocked to Some Degree, Will Exercise and Diet etc. Help Unblock Them?

There is no hard evidence that exercise, or any other measure for that matter, will help to unblock coronary arteries once atheroma has become established. Studies show that most men have at least some degree of coronary narrowing by late middle-age and this process does not appear to be reversible.

However, there is evidence that exercise and changes in diet etc. will help to prevent the *progression* of the disease. In other words, it may not make the actual narrowing any better, but there is good evidence that it will prevent it from getting any worse. In addition, since there is also evidence that regular exercise helps to increase the diameter of the coronary arteries, the amount of narrowing or atheroma may be reduced relatively by increasing the overall diameter of the artery.

Isn't the Fact that I Feel So Well at Present, a Pretty Good Guide to the State of My Health?

No it is not. Many patients who die suddenly from coronary artery disease feel perfectly well the day before. Indeed, it is remarkable how often patients will tell you that they are amazed to have suffered a heart attack, or some form of other physical illness, when just prior to the event they felt themselves to be in such robust health. Some of these misconceptions are worrying. Many people, for example, seem to think that if you suffer with hypertension (raised blood pressure) you will have severe headaches, feel generally unwell or have a whole host of other 'warning' signs. This is completely untrue. Most people with hypertension, even with quite serious elevations of their blood pressure, have no symptoms at all. Approximately 15 per cent of the adult population is thought to be hypertensive and therefore at a substantially increased risk of suffering strokes and heart disease. A raised blood cholesterol level will also not give you any symptoms. Left unchecked for a 20-year period, however, its effects could be devastating.

Many of the major disease processes only cause symptoms when they have reached a very advanced stage. Since, in most cases, the treatment for these diseases once established is unsatisfactory, it follows that the best method of dealing with them is by prevention in the first instance.

Will Running Help to Reduce the Level of My Blood Cholesterol?

Running, or any other exercise for that matter, will have very little effect, if any, on the level of your total blood cholesterol. However, as we have consistently emphasized, the level of your blood cholesterol is not the only determinant of your coronary risk. We have seen that the level of high density lipoprotein (HDL) is a better predictor of coronary events, and that the higher the level of HDL, the better the degree of protection. The desirable state of affairs, therefore, is to have a high level of HDL and a low level of total cholesterol. Exercise will not help to reduce the level of total cholesterol, but studies do suggest that exercise will increase the level of HDL. In this respect, therefore, exercise is clearly beneficial in favourably improving the blood fat profile.

I'm Nearly 60 Now, Surely I Can't Become Fit at My Age?

Provided that you are in basically sound health there is absolutely no good reason why you should not achieve a reasonable degree of cardiovascular fitness. There is a propensity in our society for regarding physical activity as the province of those individuals who are 35 years of age or younger. This is nonsense. Studies have shown that individuals in their sixties and seventies respond very favourably to training programmes and as a result can substantially improve their overall physical state. We certainly advocate that individuals in our society should be as active as possible, for as long as possible.

It would be foolish to suggest that a 70-year-old man could achieve the same kind of aerobic fitness as a man in his thirties or forties. Maximum oxygen consumption ($\dot{V}O_2$ max) decreases with age and this is independent of how much physical activity is performed. However, the authors believe that middle aged and elderly people in this country accept a standard of physical activity and fitness which is very substantially below that which they are actually capable of. It is also important to realize that in elderly people physical activity may have an important social part to play. So, the answer is, if you begin gently, and have realistic targets, via a programme of *moderate* activity, there is no reason why you should not become involved in a programme of regular activity. Indeed, we would positively encourage you to do so.

Is It True that Women Have Less Heart Disease than Men?

Until the menopause the frequency of coronary heart disease in women is approximately five or six times less than that in men. After the menopause the incidence in women rises steeply, so that by the age of 70 and above, the incidence in both sexes is approximately the same. Despite the relatively low incidence of heart disease in women prior to the menopause, it should be clearly understood that it is still the biggest overall killer in women. In addition, there is a powerful association between cigarette smoking and the contraceptive pill, which may be responsible for an increase in coronary heart disease amongst women.

Why women should have a relative degree of protection prior to the menopause is not clearly understood. It is known that levels of high density lipoprotein (HDL) tend to be higher in women, and since HDL is known to be cardio-protective, this may account for at least some of the difference in mortality rates. Whether the levels of HDL in turn are related to female hormones such as oestrogen and progesterone, has yet to be clarified.

Isn't all this Concern about the Safety of Exercise Overstated? After All, Running Is the Most Natural Form of Human Exercise and Will Have Been Practised for Virtually the Whole of Man's Span on Earth

The answer to this question is that it is the *setting* in which the exercise takes place which is the important factor. It is perfectly true that running and walking are very natural human activities and that ordinarily one would not have to be concerned about the question of risk. However, the technological revolution of the twentieth century, including the industrialization of food production, has produced the environment in which most individuals in Western society now exist. One of the direct results of these changes has been the modern epidemic of coronary heart disease, which is almost certainly the result of the changes in diet, exercise and stress that we have discussed earlier in this book. The environment in which most of us find ourselves is thus unique in human history. The fact is that running is a perfectly safe human activity *provided* that your coronary arteries are not blocked. Since blocked coronary arteries appear to be a feature of twentieth century Western society, it follows that there *are* special reasons for advocating a cautious approach when individuals, particularly those in middle age, take up exercise programmes. Safety, *must* be a paramount consideration.

I Exercised a Great Deal in my Teens and Early Twenties. Doesn't the Fact I Was Highly Active in My Youth, Afford Me Some Measure of Protection Against Heart Disease in Middle and Later Life?

It is surprising how many individuals believe that high activity patterns in early life continue to provide protection into middle life and even into old age. There is no evidence to suggest this. On the contrary, the available evidence shows quite clearly that the benefits of exercise cannot be stored and that the cardio-protective effect is only shown in those groups who *maintain* relatively high levels of physical activity. The fact that you may have been actively involved in various sporting pursuits in your school or university life does not provide you with any cardio-protective benefit in middle or later life.

What Is a 'Normal' Blood Cholesterol Level?

We have stressed the importance of blood cholesterol levels in detail elsewhere. In brief, the following comments are the most relevant. There is no such thing as a 'normal' blood cholesterol level. There is only an increasing risk of developing cardiovascular disease with increasing levels of blood cholesterol. Therefore, if your blood cholesterol is 7.5 mmol/l you are at a substantially greater risk of developing cardiovascular disease than if your blood cholesterol is 3.8 mmol/l. Most laboratories quote a normal range of between approximately 3.4 and 7.5 mmol/l. These 'normal' values, however, are based upon data obtained from a population that is being decimated by coronary heart disease. In this sense, therefore, the population cannot be regarded as a normal one and it follows that the blood cholesterol levels obtained from it cannot be regarded as 'normal' either.

There is some confusion about whether heart disease is related to high fat diets, or whether it is specifically related to high blood cholesterol. Not everyone who eats a high fat diet develops a high blood cholesterol level. Nevertheless, if your diet is high in saturated fats, there is a much greater likelihood that your blood cholesterol will be significantly elevated. In population studies where the intake of animal fats is known to be high, the tendency towards elevated blood cholesterol in that population is substantially increased. Because of this, there is not only an association between high blood cholesterol and the development of cardiac disease, but also between diets that are high in animal fats and the development of coronary disease.

Many people are confused about whether it is the level of blood cholesterol that is important or the dietary intake of animal fat. The answer is, what is relevant is the actual level of your blood cholesterol. However, since we know that diets that are high in animal fats *tend* to produce blood cholesterol levels that are higher than average, there is also an association between dietary fat intake and coronary heart disease.

If you eat a diet that is high in saturated fats and yet still have a blood cholesterol level below 4 mmol/l, then your diet is probably doing you no harm at all. If, however, that high fat diet is producing a blood cholesterol of 8 or 9 mmol/l, then it probably does matter very significantly. There is no doubt that some individuals have an innate ability to handle high animal fat and cholesterol diets without producing high levels of blood cholesterol. For these individuals there is probably no benefit in reducing their total saturated fat intake, except in so far as it will produce a substantial reduction in total calorie intake which will be useful if they are trying to lose weight.

If possible, therefore, you should arrange to have your blood cholesterol levels measured. If they are substantially above 6 or 7 mmol/l, you should definitely take some action to reduce your total saturated fat and cholesterol intake. If your blood cholesterol is between 4 and 5 mmol/l, then this is certainly acceptable. Bear in mind, however, that there is a linear relationship between levels of blood cholesterol and the probability of developing coronary heart disease. In simple terms, therefore, the best blood cholesterol is the lowest blood cholesterol.

Is Weight Training an Effective Form of Exercise?

Weight training *per se* does not produce any significant improvement in cardiovascular efficiency or performance. Weight training primarily increases strength, and unless very specialized training programmes are utilized, it does not result in a significant increase in cardiovascular

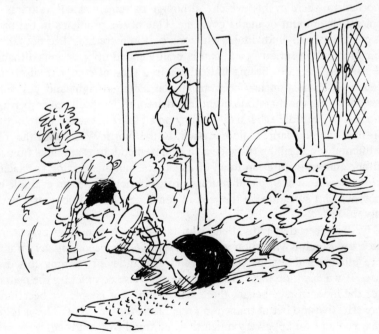

efficiency or aerobic capacity. Many individuals who lift weights regularly or use gym equipment are very surprised when they visit our laboratory to find that their aerobic capacity and their cardiovascular fitness is actually quite poor. Weight training is undoubtedly useful in promoting and maintaining muscular strength and tone, and there is certainly a place for it in the weekly training programme, but it must always be an addition to and not a substitute for an adequate programme of cardiovascular training. Most well-equipped gymnasiums these days have stationary exercise bicycles and treadmills available, so we would advise you to use these forms of exercise in combination with your regular resistance training.

Is Running a Marathon a Good Idea?

In recent years there has been a tremendous increase in interest in distance running, especially over the marathon distance of 26 miles 385 yards. Many thousands of middle-aged, hitherto sedentary individuals have found the challenge irresistible and spend many hours of their leisure time in preparation. Many thousands of people have found tremendous satisfaction and a great sense of achievement in training for, and completing the marathon distance successfully. This is entirely understandable because as an endurance event it is unparalleled.

Unfortunately, there has also been an increase in the number of deaths reported in such events which, although extremely small, attracts a tremendous amount of media coverage. One of the problems in the past has been that many individuals who took part in marathons had not taken their preparation seriously and consequently ended up in serious difficulties early in the race. Seeing individuals in a state of complete disorientation and exhaustion has been an all too common sight and has only served to bring the marathon event into disrepute. We well remember the spectacle of a middle-aged man crawling on all fours in the direction of the finishing line of a large scale marathon in the North West, with the TV commentator describing the spectacle as 'a tremendous example of human courage and an inspiration to all of us'. It was not an edifying spectacle. Neither was it an example of courage or inspiration. It was an example of ignorance and stupidity on the part of someone who had obviously been sadly misled.

The signs are that individuals who take part in marathon events, of which the London Marathon is a good example, are becoming very much more informed about the problems and difficulties of running this distance. If we examine the marathon times of those completing the course since the modern race began, there is no doubt that people are becoming more effective and better trained in preparation for the event. This is to be welcomed and we hope very much that the trend will continue.

As to how you decide whether to run a marathon is more difficult. It is an individual decision and there are a number of factors you will have to take into account. First, you will have to spend a considerable amount of time in preparation and you should think carefully about the effects on your social life, business and family commitments. Running 70 miles a week in preparation for a marathon is a large undertaking and one which you should not enter upon lightly. Secondly, you should have already achieved a good standard of cardiovascular fitness, utilizing the training programme we have outlined. You can then embark upon a more specialized training regime. If you are in basically sound health without any serious medical problems and you have achieved a reasonable standard of cardiovascular fitness, then there is no good cardiological reason why you should not prepare for and successfully complete the marathon distance.

We are extremely cautious about recommending marathon running to the individuals who attend our laboratory. This is not because we intrinsically have anything against long-distance running but because many of the individuals who attempt such distances are simply not sufficiently prepared and are inadequately informed as to the problems and potential risks involved. If you take the event seriously, plan your preparation carefully and set realistic goals, then the event can be interesting and rewarding. However, you should bear in mind that running marathon distances will not necessarily improve your health. It will almost certainly improve your aerobic capacity, up to a point, but there is no evidence that this is, in itself, cardio-protective. We have already stated clearly elsewhere, and now reiterate, there is probably no benefit, in health terms, of running 70 miles a week as opposed to 20 miles a week. The major difference in cardio-protection as a result of exercise is seen in those groups that are *moderately* active as opposed to sedentary. Most people, however, do not run marathons because they believe it will protect them from heart disease. They run the distance because they feel a sense of excitement and challenge and because they basically enjoy running.

If I Decide to Follow Your Recommendations to Give Up Cigarette Smoking, Lose Weight, Become More Physically Active, Change My Diet, Restrict My Salt Intake and Ensure My Blood Pressure Is Normal, Is there Any Guarantee I Will Live a Single Day Longer?

No: it would be absurd to suggest such a guarantee existed. All that one is entitled to claim is that there is a substantially reduced probability that you would die or suffer premature disability due to cardiovascular disease, stroke and other so-called 'Western' illnesses. It is a question of the degree of risk that you are prepared to accept; the more risk factors you have, then obviously the greater the likelihood that you will become a victim. That does not mean to say you will, merely that it is more *likely* that you will.

Is It Safe for Me to Exercise During Pregnancy?

In general terms the straightforward and simple answer to this question is 'yes'. As more women of reproductive age become involved in regular exercise it is likely that many of them will wish to continue exercising throughout their pregnancy. The natural concern, of course, is whether or not this continued exercise will have any adverse effects upon the mother and particularly upon the fetus. Pregnancy is obviously a state of intimate interaction between the mother and the foetus and everything possible must be done to maintain and to develop that interaction.

A lack of oxygen to the uterus and therefore to the fetus during pregnancy is potentially dangerous, and in theory it could be argued that if the oxygen requirements for the mother herself are sufficiently high, for example during vigorous exercise, then blood and oxygen may well be diverted from the uterus, and therefore the fetus, to serve the increased maternal requirements. Also, again theoretically, the accumulation of lactic acid and other metabolic products as a result of the mother's exercise could have a potentially harmful effect upon the developing fetus. Finally, the well-being of the baby and the eventual outcome of the birth could well be influenced by repetitive mechanical stress on the developing uterus and on the mother's skeletal and soft tissues. As pregnancy advances therefore, there is at least a potential hazard to be taken into account.

The first thing to note is that there is a tremendous advantage to be gained from being physically fit at the commencement of pregnancy. A healthy cardiovascular system and a good standard of overall muscle tone would serve the mother well throughout the duration of the pregnancy and during the birth itself. During the early months of pregnancy many women find that nausea and sickness preclude their continuing with their normal exercise programmes. So in the first three months they may well discontinue exercise and many of them never take it up again during the duration of the pregnancy. As pregnancy progresses fewer women will continue to exercise, and in those that do their exercise capacity falls substantially. Nausea, vomiting, fatigue, joint pain, ligament pain, back pain and uterine contractions, and also fear of harm to the infant, are all factors that tend to reduce the exercise component as pregnancy advances.

To date there is no evidence that continued exercise throughout pregnancy, even to within a few days of delivery, will, in itself, have any deleterious effect upon mother or baby. Indeed in some studies the complications of labour and delivery were less pronounced in those who continued to exercise during pregnancy than in their non-exercising counterparts. So the message is fairly clear, if you are already involved in exercise prior to your pregnancy there is no good reason why you should not continue to exercise throughout its duration. This, of course, assumes that symptoms such as nausea, vomiting and discomfort do not prevent your exercising. If you are running, then you should recognize that the actual mechanical problems of exercise will increase as the pregnancy proceeds. If you think that running is no longer comfortable, then swimming or the use of a stationary exercise bicycle are very suitable alternatives.

This is such an individual matter that it is only possible to make broad, general statements. There are some common-sense factors which must be taken into account. An obvious example is that if you are eight months pregnant, a fall whilst you are attempting to run could be extremely serious. Therefore, unless you are a very experienced runner, we suggest that as the pregnancy progresses you move towards swimming or the use of a stationary exercise bicycle.

We would not recommend that you should start a running programme during pregnancy. There is no hard evidence to suggest that this is especially dangerous, but given the fact that it will place very considerable demands upon an untrained cardiovascular system it could have a potentially adverse effect upon the developing fetus. We would suggest that gentle swimming or the use of a stationary exercise bicycle are more appropriate to first-time exercisers in pregnancy because in both these activities the weight is supported and the demand upon the heart and lungs is therefore less. We also strongly recommend that you should attend any available ante-natal exercise classes as they can be of enormous benefit in teaching appropriate breathing exercises and improving abdominal tone.

We believe that if you maintain your fitness throughout pregnancy with mild exercise you will find the delivery easier and you will recover in a shorter period of time.

When the pregnancy is over there will need to be a period of rest to allow the uterus to return to its normal state. Vigorous exercise during this period would be unwise, but brisk walking and similar forms of exercise should be encouraged and taken up almost immediately. In summary:

- There is no evidence that moderate exercise during pregnancy will have any harmful effect upon mother or baby. Indeed, we believe it to be beneficial.
- Achieving physical fitness prior to pregnancy is an excellent investment.
- Exercise will inevitably become harder as pregnancy progresses

and you should accept the increase in fatigue as an entirely normal phenomenon.

- If exercise during pregnancy causes you to feel unwell or you experience any discomfort you should stop.

What Effect Does Exercise Have Upon the Menstrual Cycle?

During the past five years or so a number of published studies have shown a relatively high incidence of menstrual cycle irregularities in athletes. Evidence suggests that sustained exercise stimulates marked changes in the menstrual cycle, although it is not yet fully understood how these changes occur. As more women participate in sporting and recreational activities, the incidence of menstrual cycle irregularities will increase. Most of the data available have been obtained from studies in Olympic gymnasts, swimmers, track and field participants, basketball players, marathon runners and recreational runners. Among the factors contributing to the menstrual cycle disturbance are weight loss and changes in hormonal secretion.

Two major forms of menstrual cycle disturbance occur: *oligomenorrhoea*, when the menstrual period is scanty and there is only a very small amount of blood loss and *amenorrhoea*, when the periods stop altogether and the woman may become infertile. The incidence of such abnormalities varies enormously and can range between seven and 100 per cent depending upon how menstrual cycle disturbances are classified. However, when only oligomenorrhoea or amenorrhoea are considered, the figures range from seven to 43 per cent.

Although the incidence of the abnormalities varies so widely, it does appear that a major factor is the total energy expenditure during training. The highest incidence of menstrual cycle irregularities occurs in those subjects who train the most. For example, some studies have shown that in runners who accummulate less than 20 miles a week, the incidence of amenorrhoea was 8 per cent. As soon as the training mileage increased above 20 miles a week there was a pronounced increase in amenorrhoea to 20 per cent. Thereafter the figures increased proportionately, with increased training mileage, so that for women who ran 80 miles a week or more the incidence was 43 per cent.

Given that such disturbances in the menstrual cycle are so common, and are likely to increase as more women participate in sport and recreational activities, we should ask if there is any need for concern. In general there is not, and if your menstrual cycle does change as a result of exercise this need not concern you unduly. Menstrual function reverts to normal within one or two months in most women when exercise ceases. In addition, we should remember that although regular strenuous exercise can cause menstrual dysfunction, there are many other factors that may also be associated with oligo- or amenorrhoea and thus increase a woman's susceptibility to this condition. Low body weight and low body fat are most commonly associated with exercise-related menstrual disturbances, but other factors, including emotional stress and dietary changes, may also be important. In many women the combined effects of two or more stresses as well as strenuous exercise may cause disruption in the normal menstrual cycle.

It is evident, therefore, that menstrual cycle disturbances are common, but usually revert to normal on cessation of exercise. If you are involved in high levels of physical activity, you may well become amenorrhoeic and if so it is obvious that your chances of becoming pregnant are remote. However, cessation of exercise or even reduction in intensity of exercise should return your menstrual cycle to normal. One word of caution: the fact that you may be amenorrhoeic does not exclude the possibility of your becoming pregnant. Some amenorrhoeic athletes have become pregnant without having menstruated for several months. In other words, regular running is not a reliable method of contraception!

Some individuals note a reduction in their exercise performance as a result of taking the contraceptive pill. The reasons for this are not clear but it may be due to the effects of progesterone. It usually manifests itself as a slight increase in breathlessness but this does appear to moderate and eventually disappear with the passage of time. More work needs to be done in this area, but if you notice this yourself, you should be reassured that it is likely to be only a temporary phenomenon.

Heart Disease Is the Biggest Killer in Men: What Are the Biggest Preventable Causes of Death in Women?

Heart disease is the biggest killer in men and is *overall* the biggest killer in women; however, as we have seen previously, the incidence of coronary heart disease in the pre-menopausal period is low and it is only after the menopause that the incidence of heart disease in women rises substantially. The major cause of premature disability and death in younger, i.e. pre-menopausal females, are various forms of cancer, especially cancer of the cervix and of the breast. Since we are not fully familiar with the mechanisms which lead to either of these conditions (although there is some evidence that cancer of the breast may be related to high fat diets, but this is not yet proved), it is not possible to give any guidelines as to *actual prevention*. However, the *early identification* of these diseases is of the utmost importance because various studies have shown that subsequent morbidity and mortality rates can be substantially reduced by early diagnosis.

Screening for cervical cancer is especially important, as approximately 2,000 women in England and Wales die each year from this form of cancer (the 1984 figure being 1,917). Regular examination using the cervical smear is very important as an early means of detecting this condition. The present guidelines with regard to the frequency of this examination are somewhat varied, in some areas it is three years and in others five. Present evidence would suggest that this is inadequate. We recommend a cervical smear on every sexually active woman over the age of 20 on an annual basis (some work has even suggested this should be on a six-monthly basis).

Breast cancer was responsible for the deaths of 13,310 women in England and Wales in 1984. Regular self-examination by palpation of the breasts and mammography could result in a substantial reduction of this mortality rate. Mammography is a specialized technique in which the breast is X-rayed using standardized views. Controlled trials in Sweden and New York have shown reductions in mortality from breast cancer of between 30 and 40 per cent as a result of this form of screening. Mammography is not widely available to the general public but where it is available the recommendations are now fairly clear. The accepted standard on good practice is that suggested by the American College of Radiologists. They recommend that routine mammography should be performed between the ages of 35 and 40 and that subsequent mammographic examinations should be performed at one- to three-yearly intervals. After the age of 50 an annual examination is recommended.

A regular cervical smear is something you should be able to obtain fairly easily and if mammography facilities are not available then it is certainly important you should examine your own breasts regularly for any abnormal lumps. If you are in any way concerned, then you should, of course, see your own general practitioner.

What About Alcohol Consumption? Are There Any Useful Guidelines for Safe Drinking?

As a nation we are drinking far too much for our own good and the national consumption of alcohol has increased dramatically since the Second World War; the whole of Europe, in fact, is drinking more than it used to. Between 1962 and 1982 wine drinking in this country increased by 240 per cent, spirit drinking increased 95 per cent and beer drinking was up by 22 per cent. Moreover, we are being actively encouraged to drink even more. The alcohol industry in 1981 spent an estimated £100 million on advertising.

It is therefore hardly surprising that alcohol abuse is now a major health problem which is increasingly affecting the younger age groups. The number of deaths caused by alcohol is unknown; nor can we quantify the full extent of the social and human costs of alcohol abuse. In England and Wales it is estimated that there are 750,000 to 1,000,000 people with serious alcohol problems, but the number may be considerably higher. Between 1970 and 1980 deaths from alcoholic liver disease increased by just over 60 per cent. As a rough estimate, alcohol abuse in England and Wales in 1981 probably cost in excess of £1,000 million (this includes the cost of health services, police and prison, alcohol-related road accidents and loss of industrial output). Without question, therefore, alcohol abuse represents a major economic, social and human problem.

What effects can alcohol have on the body?

The active ingredient in all alcoholic drinks is a substance called ethyl-alcohol. It is this that causes changes in mood and behaviour and which, in excess, can cause serious health problems. Some drinks, spirits for example, contain more alcohol per unit volume but, of course, we tend to drink these in smaller measures.

Alcohol is removed from the bloodstream by the liver. Bubbly or diluted drinks (for example, champagne or gin with lots of tonic) enter the blood more quickly and therefore tend to produce rapid effects. Alcohol exerts its harmful effects in a number of ways and there is virtually no system or organ in the body that cannot be damaged in some way by alcohol. It can produce anything from simple nausea to a rare but lethal form of brain damage called 'Chianti drinker's syndrome'.

In the liver alcohol can cause the normal liver cells to be replaced by fat and later by fibrous scar tissue (cirrhosis). It can also cause obesity and vitamin deficiency. It can worsen elevated blood pressure and by a direct toxic effect upon the heart muscle (a cardiomyopathy) it may produce heart failure. Excess alcohol can cause a variety of forms of brain damage and serious neurological problems. It may also cause damage to the stomach and intestines and excess alcohol consumption is associated with an increased incidence of cancer of the mouth, throat and liver. It may cause a wide range of psychiatric disorders, sexual difficulties and depression.

It is also important to note that women are physically more vulnerable to the effects of alcohol. Alcohol circulating around the body is distributed throughout the body's fluid. In men, this constitutes between 55 and 65 per cent of the body but in women only 45 to 55 per cent. Therefore, since the body fluid is proportionately less in women, the alcohol concentration tends to be higher. Women tend to have smaller bodies than men, so again the alcohol is more concentrated. Moreover, women also tend to have smaller livers and are therefore more likely to do them damage at lower levels of drinking. Drinking in pregnancy is potentially hazardous. Everything a pregnant woman drinks the fetus drinks too and the effect on the developing baby is much greater because it is so small. Some research has suggested the birth weight of a baby might be reduced by an alcohol intake of as little as ten units (see below) per week, and although this is controversial, there is a general consensus that the lower the alcohol consumption during pregnancy, the better. In very heavy drinking during pregnancy the child may be born with the fetal alcohol syndrome (FAS), in which the baby is born with facial and physical deformities. The baby may also be mentally retarded and growth and development in general are usually slower than normal.

So how much alcohol is safe?

One of the difficulties in suggesting safe levels of alcohol consumption for both men and women is that there is an enormous individual variation in response to similar quantities of alcohol. In addition, there is relatively little information on which to base recommendations for safe drinking; different studies have produced different suggestions. What is clear, however, is that the more you drink, the more likely you are to damage your health.

It is useful to quantify alcohol consumption in terms of standard units, thus:

    1 standard unit = 1 half pint of beer
                      1 single sherry, vermouth etc.
                      1 single spirit, whisky etc.
                      1 glass of wine

Thus, if you drink two pints of beer and one gin and tonic, you will have consumed a total of five units. If you did this seven nights a week, your weekly consumption would be 35 units. Using this as a simple guide, you should be able to obtain a rough estimate of your weekly consumption of alcohol. The following should enable you to set this consumption in context:

1 Men, 51 units per week or more: women, 36 units per week or more. At this level of drinking you run the risk of serious damage to your health and you should do everything possible to moderate your alcohol intake substantially.

2 Men, 37–50 units per week: women, 25–35 units per week. You are creeping up to the level where damage to your health becomes highly probable. Your drinking may also lead you into social and legal difficulties and you should think very carefully about whether you want to continue drinking at this level.

3 Men, 21–36 units per week: women, 14–24 units per week. If you spread out this sort of alcohol consumption throughout the week

you are very unlikely to have any long-term health damage. However, concentrating this total consumption into one or two drinking episodes could increase your chances of having an accident or suffering ill-health.

4 Men, up to 20 units per week: women, up to 13 units per week. Drinking at this level carries no long-term health risk. Indeed, the health educational council recommends 20 and 13 units for men and women respectively as a sensible drinking level.

So far as drinking and driving is concerned, the best advice is clearly if you drink, don't drive. As a rough guide a man who has drunk five units of alcohol (two and a half pints of beer) and a women who has drunk three units of alcohol will both be at the legal limit. It takes about one hour for the body to rid itself of one standard drink (one unit), so if you drink a lot at lunchtime you could still be well over the limit by the evening.

By keeping a close eye on your total alcohol consumption throughout the week it should be reasonably easy to maintain this within fairly safe limits. It is also useful to have two or three days per week without any drink at all and also to limit yourself to a certain number of drinks per day. Drinking in 'rounds' with groups of people tends to make you drink more than you would otherwise, and so this is something to avoid. It is also useful to make your first drink of the evening a long, soft drink which will quench your thirst before you start drinking alcohol.

Thinking in standard units of alcohol is a useful means of assessing your approximate alcohol intake. Some forms of alcohol, however, are not easy to quantify in standard units. For example, if someone gives you a bottle of Polish vodka or Japanese saki for your birthday how can you assess how many units of alcohol each of these drinks contains? In Britain the matter is further complicated, for you may find any one of three measures for alcohol content on a label. One is original gravity (OG) – a measure of the quantity of certain ingredients used in making beer. The second is degrees proof – a very old method of measuring alcohol content (using gunpowder!) and the third is per cent alcohol – a measure of the proportion of alcohol in a given quantity of drink. This label actually allows you to work out fairly easily the number of units of alcohol in non-standard strength drinks. For example, as a very rough guide:

1 half pint of 4% beer = 1 unit
1 half pint of 8% beer = 2 units

1 glass of 12% wine = 1 unit
1 glass of 15% wine = $1\frac{1}{4}$ units

1 single measure of 20% fortified wine = 1 unit
1 single measure of 25% fortified wine = $1\frac{1}{4}$ units

1 single measure of 40% spirit $=$ 1 unit
1 single measure of 50% spirit $=$ $1\frac{1}{4}$ units.

The European Commission has proposed that all alcohol should be labelled with percentage alcohol content. This form of labelling would clearly be an advantage.

Some myths about alcohol are worth considering. A common one is that drinking beer is less harmful than drinking wine or spirits. In fact, unit for unit, alcoholic drinks are all as potentially harmful. We have already seen that one standard measure of whisky contains the same amount of alcohol as half a pint of beer. It is simply a question of how many units of alcohol you take and not necessarily the form in which you take them.

Another common myth is that alcohol is a stimulant. The reverse is in fact true; alcohol is actually a depressant. It may help you to lose your inhibitions and give you the impression that it has a stimulant effect, but it only achieves this because it dulls the higher centres in the brain.

Some people also believe that the absence of a hangover is reassuring; in other words, you are more likely to get a hangover the more you drink. However, some people rarely get hangovers and others may get one after only one or two drinks. It is perfectly possible to be doing yourself serious damage and not have a hangover at all.

Finally, despite all that has been said, not all alcohol is bad for you. Indeed moderate amounts of alcohol taken regularly may exert a potentially beneficial effect on the heart. Also, of course, drinking is a very enjoyable and social activity and can be a source of humour and relaxation. As with everything else, it is simply a question of degree; you must use alcohol properly and recognize its potential hazards.

11

How to Die Young as Late as Possible

If we are to see any substantial change in the health of the population during the next decade or so, we shall need to take urgent and concerted action to do something *now*. The enormity of the problems we face can no longer be left unchallenged and we have to recognize that our efforts at dealing with them have, thus far at least, been woefully inadequate.

How can we remain so complacent in the face of such an unremitting threat to the health of so many members of the population? Perhaps like the threat of nuclear war, it is another example of the 'ostrich syndrome'. Burying your head in the sand will not make the problem go away, but at least you are not faced with the psychological consequences of confronting it. We have to face up to the fact that most of our burden of disease, including coronary and other forms of cardiovascular disease, diseases of the bowel, diabetes, gallstones etc. and also cancer, are at least potentially preventable. Indeed, so far as cancer is concerned, the growing body of evidence would suggest that there is almost as much information to be communicated about cancer prevention as there is about preventing coronary heart disease and other so-called, 'Western diseases'. When Doll and Peto produced their review on 'The causes of cancer' for the American Congressional Office of Technology Assessment in 1981, they concluded that between 80 and 90 per cent of all cancers could, in principle, be avoided.

The challenge of prevention for heart disease, strokes, cancer and other Western diseases remains largely unanswered, and yet it remains perhaps the greatest medical challenge of our generation. To begin to meet this challenge we shall need to effect a significant change in attitudes amongst doctors and other health professionals as well as in the lay public whom they serve.

A change in the attitude of doctors and other health professionals

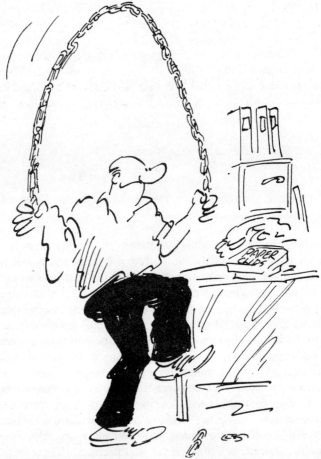

towards the concept of prevention is a prerequisite if a concerted and coordinated programme is to be implemented. There are, however, major problems in this direction, not the least of which is the fact that most doctors undergo very little, if any, training in preventive medicine. In addition, most doctors have the most rudimentary knowledge of nutrition and can hardly be expected to advise others. Without question much more emphasis needs to be placed on the concept of prevention, including the principles of nutrition, in the basic training given in our medical schools. The perception of preventive medicine as being a 'Cinderella' specialty must change; in fact, it must assume a primary role.

At the present time our medical training tends to conform to what we call the 'disease' model. This view of illness and disease pictures the body as a complex machine which, when diseased or damaged in any way, will provide a recognizable pattern of symptoms. The doctor then addresses himself to these symptoms and provides the appropriate treatment. At the outset, therefore, the doctor is interested not in health, but in disease and in the symptoms that disease provides. This is why, as we have said before, at the present time we do not have a National Health Service, but a 'National Disease Service'. This symptom-orientated concept is a passive one – we sit and wait until the body becomes diseased and then attempt to treat it. But in the case of heart disease, once a condition has been established it is extremely difficult to treat effectively. Previously it may have been appropriate to adopt a symptom-orientated approach to illness because we did not have a basic knowledge of the causes of many diseases, but large scale research programmes during the past two decades have yielded an enormous amount of data upon which we can now base an effective programme for disease prevention, particularly in relation to coronary heart disease and other forms of cardiovascular disease. This body of knowledge is growing all the time and so we shall be able to refine our programmes as our knowledge base grows. What is clear, however, is that we no longer have any excuse to remain acquiescent and inactive. We have to move away from a passive, symptom-orientated approach towards an active, enthusiastic and well-informed attempted at prevention.

The lay public also will need to change its attitude towards disease and towards the doctors and other health professionals to whom they look for guidance. First, we have to show people that health and well-being for them and for their families is not simply a question of good luck. It can be achieved and maintained by the application of fairly simple principles provided they are given access to the appropriate information. Secondly, we have to emphasize that health and well-being are not the sole responsibility of the family doctor, and whilst, without question, modern medicine could do much to help us when we do become ill, we should not rely upon them as a first line of defence. We must also learn to leave without a prescription when we visit our general practitioner and to encourage the doctor himself not to feel guilty because he has not provided one. This situation is clearly absurd and we must be more rigorous, both in our prescribing and in the use of the drugs which are available. When the heath professionals have placed the responsibility for health primarily with the individual, they must then provide him with the necessary information to achieve and maintain a good standard of health and fitness. Information with regard to exercise, proper nutrition etc. needs to be available and it is encouraging that recent television programmes and press articles have been placing a great deal of emphasis on correct eating. Exercise has also become popular, although in many cases for the wrong reasons.

If we are to talk in terms of prevention, there is no more important place to begin this process than in the schools. Children are remarkably perceptive and receptive towards matters which concern their health and well-being and our own experience suggests that they are able to assimilate this information remarkably effectively and quickly. Coronary heart disease has a long incubation. It starts in young children; if one looks at the arteries of even very young children who have died from other causes the fatty infiltration or 'plaque' formation in the coronary and other arteries is already evident. Correct nutrition must be implemented at an early stage and recognition of high risk individuals is equally as important in children as it is in adults. At the present time we do not have any effective screening programme for high risk individuals in our schools and even though it is evident that the wisest course of action is to act before the process of coronary heart disease becomes fixed and irreversible. If we are to alter lifestyles and behaviour patterns effectively, then the best time to accomplish this is before patterns and habits of behaviour are firmly entrenched, i.e. in childhood.

We believe that, if possible, correct nutrition, exercise and lifestyles should be fostered before the age of 15 or 16. This is because between the ages of 16 and 35 years it is difficult to change established patterns of behaviour. This period of young adult life is known as the era of 'immortality', that is to say that during this period the individual perceives illness and death as something which happens to other people. He may smoke cigarettes or take little exercise but because he feels himself to be well, he does not consciously think of the effects these habits may be having upon his system or upon his future health prospects.

The age of immortality – between 16 and 35 – is a long period and also a critical one. It is therefore important to induce behaviour patterns in early childhood that will be carried on through the early years of adult life into mid and later life. There could be no better forum for achieving this than the classroom. And yet, thus far, we have conspicuously failed to act to implement such programmes. Many children come from families where there is a high incidence of unexplained cardiac death. This is often because there is a genetic tendency within that family group towards having a very high blood cholesterol level, high blood pressure or some other major coronary risk factor. Yet not even the children of these high risk families are effectively identified and managed. This means that if a child of ten has a blood cholesterol of 15 or 20 mmol/l this is likely to remain undetected for most of his life and the first and only manifestation of that abnormality may be when he presents in middle life with symptoms of angina or even sudden cardiac death.

We cannot any longer be complacent about such issues or choose to disregard them because they are not convenient. We *can* mount effective and comprehensive screening programmes in schools provided we have the will to do so. The resources must be found, but the will to act must be apparent. The actual setting up of the programmes is simply a question of

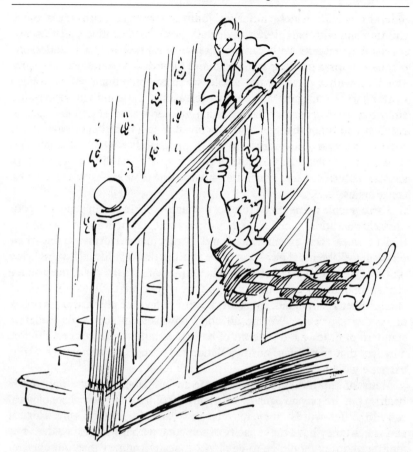

'engineering'. If we choose, once again, to do nothing, then in 20–30 years from now these 'at risk' children will become the cardiac victims of the next generation.

Regular exercise, the effective identification and management of hypertension, the control of smoking habits, the effective application of the basic principles of nutrition etc. when applied in combination, can and will have a major impact upon the health of the population. We believe that during the next decade or two there will be a growing awareness among the general population that preventive medicine *can* deliver the goods in the same way that it has already begun to do so in the USA and certain European countries.

We have emphasized the role of exercise in health maintenance because while it is only one among a number of factors, we have shown that there are reasons for considering it to be of major importance. During the past five to ten years or so we have prescribed exercise to literally thousands of individuals with widely differing abilities. Working with spina bifida children and with paraplegics, sedentary business executives, professional sportsmen, patients with cardiac disease or those who have undergone coronary bypass grafting and world and Olympic class athletes, has provided us with a view of the whole spectrum of human activity. Each working day in our laboratory convinces us that those individuals who are almost entirely sedentary have a much greater risk of developing cardiovascular and other diseases. But it is not simply a question of being more prone to disease and premature death or disability which characterizes these individuals; many of them have a quality of life which is very substantially below that which they are capable of, and it is this which also concerns us.

These people do not need to be overweight, feeble and in generally poor physical condition. Neither do they often appreciate that there is a connection between their psychological and intellectual performance and their physical well-being. They seem to be drifting through life as it were firing on two cylinders instead of four. The unpleasant truth is that the average British male is an extremely poor physical specimen. Watching a world class runner is a magnificent sight, but it is a level of physical activity few of us can aspire to. We are all able, however, to achieve a moderate standard of fitness, and in terms of basic health this is all we need aim for. The fact that so many of our population fail even to attempt such a step is extremely disturbing.

Many of the individuals who come to our laboratory are apparently healthy but are physiologically substantially older than their chronological age. In other words, they may be 35 years old, but on physiological assessment they have the capacity of someone perhaps 20 years older. The aim for all of us should be to be physiologically younger than our chronological age. Occasionally we see cases of this; we see 60-year-olds or even those in their early seventies who have the physiological capacity of men ten or 20 years younger. Watching a 65-year-old man exercising with a capacity equivalent to that of most 25- or 30-year-olds is very encouraging indeed, and there is no question that those individuals, even in their fifties, sixties and seventies, who have been exercising habitually for most of their lives have a physiological capacity greater than their chronological age would suggest and in general they tend to be healthier and fitter than their non-exercising counterparts.

It is for this reason that we profoundly believe exercise can help to retard the ageing process. What we mean by this is *not* that you will necessarily live longer, but you will be much less likely to die or be disabled prematurely by cardiovascular disease, cancer or another of the 'Western diseases'. In this sense you may well be able to achieve more than the allotted three score years and ten. However, this is not primarily what we mean when we talk about retarding the ageing process. Because exercise allows you to remain active for a much greater proportion of your total lifespan, even if you are to die at the age of 70 or 75, you may remain in perfect health into your late sixties or even your early seventies. In other words, you will be 'old' for a relatively short period of time.

If old age is marked by declining activity and poor health, then many of the individuals who attend our laboratory in their fifties or even their early forties have already entered that period of life. This is a sad comment on our attitude towards our health and a reflection on how sedentary life-styles, combined with poor nutrition etc., can have a catastrophic effect upon our quality of life and our future health prospects. In our experience, a sedentary lifestyle means that the ageing process, which is marked by decreased physical activity and failing health, tends to affect individuals much earlier. Because exercise helps to retard this process, you remain active for much longer, your quality of life is immeasurably better and although you must eventually die, you can at least die young as late as possible!

Conclusions

The points we have discussed in this book can be summarized in the following check-list:

- Make *time* to look after your health.
- Keep your weight within reasonable limits.
- If you are a cigarette smoker, give up immediately.
- If you must smoke, smoke cigars or a pipe and keep your consumption to a minimum.
- Have your blood lipids (fats) particularly your cholesterol, checked.
- Have your blood pressure checked regularly.
- Reduce your salt intake.
- Where possible adhere to a low fat, high fibre diet.
- If your cholesterol is elevated, pay particular attention to your fat consumption.
- Learn to read food labels; become interested in nutrition.
- Try to educate your children about the importance of correct eating and exercise.
- Keep an eye on your alcohol consumption.
- Try to become involved in regular physical exercise, which in practice means three or four 20 or 30 minute sessions per week.
- If you are a woman, make sure you have cervical smears performed

regularly (preferably annually) and if possible regular mammography; you should certainly palpate your own breasts regularly and attend your own general practitioner if you are concerned.

- Do not become *obsessional* about any of the above.

Why Exercise?

If you have read this book you should have become convinced of the power of exercise. If you have, we have achieved our aim. The evidence is compelling; the goals are achievable and well worth achieving, so do not delay a moment longer. It may be the most important decision of your life.

Appendix 1

The Fat Problem

The following will provide a good working knowledge for those interested in a fuller explanation of the fat problem. We repeat, however, that the most important thing is that you should *act* in some way to improve your diet where possible. It is preferable that you accept a simplistic explanation of the facts and do something active, rather than be fully informed and take no action.

Cholesterol

Although cholesterol is generally regarded as the villain of the piece, it is in fact a vital component of the cells of the body, without which life could not continue. Chemically, cholesterol resembles an alcohol and is a member of a group of substances referred to as sterols. It is found only in animal products. Although it may share some of the chemical properties of fats, it is not actually a fat at all. Cholesterol is a vital constituent in the synthesis of many important substances in the body, including various hormones and the bile salts.

In addition, it is important to understand that the body makes its own cholesterol, a process which can probably occur in almost every organ throughout the body except the adult brain. The majority of cholesterol synthesis, however, is carried out in the liver, which is capable of producing many times more cholesterol than that which is obtained through the normal diet. In fact, there is an inverse relationship between the amount of cholesterol taken in the food and the amount produced by the liver, i.e. the more cholesterol you take in your food, the less the liver produces. There is presumably a mechanism capable of switching off production in the liver when the dietary cholesterol exceeds a certain level.

Why then should it be regarded as an undesirable or even dangerous substance in certain circumstances? We now know, from a vast amount of data collected in numerous studies over many years, that there is a clear relationship between cholesterol and heart disease. Few people would now dispute this association, or that the relationship is a linear one, i.e. the higher your cholesterol, the greater the risk of developing heart disease. However, it is not necessarily the level of blood cholesterol *per se* which determines the risk, but rather the form in which the cholesterol is carried.

Essentially, cholesterol does not circulate freely in the bloodstream because, like fats with which it has certain chemical properties in common, cholesterol is not soluble in liquid. Instead, it is transported around the body in association with proteins and other substances called triglycerides. The combination of protein, triglyceride and cholesterol is called a lipoprotein. There are four main groups (or fractions) of lipoproteins, which vary according to the relative amounts of triglyceride, cholesterol, protein and phospholipid in each. If we spin a sample of blood at very high speed in a centrifuge, these four fractions can be separated according to their relative density; they are known as chylomicrons, very low density lipoprotein (VLDL), low density lipoprotein (LDL) and high density lipoprotein (HDL). Each of these four fractions is made up of lipoproteins that have different densities according to the relative amounts of choles-

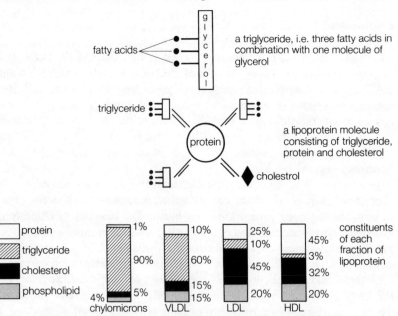

Figure A1.1   The lipoproteins.

terol, triglyceride and protein. Triglycerides are made up of three molecules of fatty acid and one molecule of glycerol (see figure A1.1).

Summarizing thus far, cholesterol is carried in the blood in four main forms of lipoproteins, VLDL, LDL, HDL and chylomicrons. Each of these lipoproteins is made up of varying amounts of cholesterol, protein and triglycerides. Remember, however, that when the blood cholesterol is measured in the body, it refers to the total cholesterol in all four groups of lipoproteins. This is important, because, as we shall see later, not all forms of cholesterol are detrimental to health – indeed some forms may be beneficial in terms of providing some degree of protection from cardiac disease.

It is clear from figure A1.1 that the major carrier of cholesterol in the bloodstream is low density lipoprotein (LDL). Very low density lipoprotein (VLDL) also contains a small amount of cholesterol, but in the main it is the major transport system for triglycerides, as are the chylomicron particles. High density lipoprotein contains relatively small amounts of both cholesterol and triglycerides.

If we take a sample of blood and measure the total amount of cholesterol it will only tell us whether the level is normal or raised. In particular, if the level is high, it will not tell us which of the four fractions is elevated. It is still a useful guide, however, and if it is abnormal, we then proceed to measure the different lipoprotein fractions to determine which is abnormal. In practice, most laboratories now measure the total cholesterol and the various lipoprotein sub-fractions automatically.

In clinical terms, we are able to label the different abnormalities in the fat profile as the hyperlipidaemias or hyperlipoproteinaemias. There are a number of different kinds, but for the purposes of this discussion only three occur with sufficient regularity to merit discussion. They are, Type 2A and Type 2B and Type 4.

Type 2A

In this group the total cholesterol is raised and when the various sub-fractions are measured, the LDL fraction is found to be increased. One would obviously expect the cholesterol level to be high, since we have seen that LDL is a major transport system for cholesterol. The triglyceride levels are normal. Subjects with a Type 2A hyperlipidaemia are very much more prone to developing heart disease, as we shall see later.

Type 2B

In this group both the LDL and the VLDL sub-fractions are increased. It is evident, therefore, that both the cholesterol and the triglyceride levels are increased (VLDL is the major transport form for triglycerides). This group is also much more likely to develop heart disease.

Type 4

This group has an increased triglyceride level (VLDL), but the cholesterol level is normal. There is evidence that those subjects who have increased levels of triglycerides may also have an increased risk of developing heart disease, although the evidence is in general not as conclusive as in those subjects who have increased levels of cholesterol. In the main, therefore, it is the level of cholesterol and in particular the level of LDL which is the important factor in any one individual. Thus the real culprit in heart disease is not cholesterol *per se*, but rather the lipoprotein sub-group known as LDL. We do not yet understand the precise mechanism whereby LDL causes the deposition of cholesterol and other fats in the lining of the artery, but there is little doubt that LDL has a major part to play in the process.

HDL (High Density Lipoprotein)

We have left discussion of HDL until this point because high density lipoprotein appears to have a vital part to play in providing a degree of *protection* from heart disease. A large amount of evidence is now available, suggesting that the level of HDL in the blood is of great importance in determining the risk of developing coronary heart disease. Indeed some workers now believe that the level of HDL may be more important than the levels of cholesterol in the LDL fraction. Evidence from the Framingham, Massachusetts, heart study has shifted attention from cholesterol levels towards levels of HDL.

The Framingham study was initiated in 1948 when the Public Health Service in the USA began a comprehensive study of heart disease in an attempt to define those factors important in its causation. A sample of the adult population was observed for more than 30 years and levels of cholesterol, HDL and other lipid sub-fractions determined. From this accumulating data it has become clear that HDL is a powerful predictor of the development of heart disease. The detail of this and other major studies need not concern us here; suffice it to say that a high level of HDL is beneficial, whilst a low level is accompanied by an increased risk of developing coronary heart disease.

HDL levels are known to be higher in women than in men and this may help to explain why there is such a difference in the incidence of heart disease between the sexes, the incidence in women being on average six times lower than in men. Whether these high levels of HDL are mediated by female hormones is not clear.

Obesity, diabetes mellitus and chronic kidney disease are all associated with low levels of HDL, and a concomitantly higher incidence of heart disease. It is also known that exercise can increase HDL levels and this mechanism may be fundamental to the protective effect exercise is known to have against heart disease.

A last point will no doubt prove a comfort to some readers who enjoy a little alcohol from time to time. HDL levels are increased by regular, moderate doses of alcohol, and as a result, the risk of coronary heart disease is decreased. However, before you rush out to your nearest public house, you should bear in mind that heavier doses of alcohol may have detrimental effects in other areas, so it would be unwise to advocate the mass prescription of large amounts of alcohol to the population as a whole.

Cholesterol: HDL Ratio

Because it is believed that the likelihood of developing heart disease is to some extent related to the level of cholesterol and HDL in the blood, it is useful to express a relationship between these sub-fractions to give some idea of the overall risk. We have seen that the higher the level of cholesterol (usually in the form of LDL), the higher the risk of heart disease; and the higher the level of HDL, the *lower* the risk of heart disease. When we express these two parameters in relation to each other we can derive something called the 'coronary heart disease risk ratio'. It is derived by dividing the total cholesterol by the HDL, i.e.

$$\frac{\text{Total cholesterol}}{\text{HDL}} = \text{Coronary heart disease risk ratio}$$

We have already mentioned that the most important question is not what the level of cholesterol is, but in what form it is carried. If your blood cholesterol is slightly raised, it may not necessarily be harmful, because if a substantial amount were carried in the HDL sub-fraction which is thought to be protective against coronary atheroma, it would clearly be an advantage. For example if your total cholesterol is 6 mmol/l and your HDL is 2 mmol/l, then your coronary heart disease risk ratio (CHDR) will be:

$$\frac{6}{2} = 3$$

which is below average, and therefore a distinct advantage. If, however, your blood cholesterol is 6 mmol/l and is mainly carried in the LDL fraction, with only a small amount (say 0.8 mmol/l) carried in the form of HDL, then the equation will look like this:

$$\frac{6}{0.8} = 7.5$$

which is above average, and would tend to place you at increased risk. The average CHDR ratio is about 5.

If we now take an example where the level of cholesterol in the blood is very high, say 12 mmol/l, and when we measure the sub-fractions we find that the level of HDL is low, e.g. 0.7 mmol/l, the CHDR ratio is:

$$\frac{12}{0.7} = 17$$

which is clearly very high, and on present evidence would place the individual at a substantially greater risk of developing problems.

These examples are meant only to illustrate that if the total cholesterol is high, it is important to know in what form it is being carried, i.e. either LDL or HDL. In practice, if your cholesterol is substantially elevated it is likely that most will be carried in the form of LDL, since it is unusual for HDL to rise much above 2 mmol/l, whereas it is quite possible for LDL cholesterol to be as high as 15 or 20 mmol/l. It is possible to manipulate both the cholesterol and the HDL fractions of the blood in a manner that will tend to improve the CHDR ratio. It is also possible to lower raised triglyceride levels which occur in Type 2B and Type 4 hyperlipidaemias (Type 2B having increased levels of triglyceride only).

Appendix 2

Personal Questionnaire
Assessment of Type A Personality, Stress and
Coping Skills

For each of the questions over, please indicate whether the item is true for
you or not by circling YES (if it applies) or NO (if it does not). We realise
that you may have reservations about a clear-cut YES or NO, but we
would like you to indicate which comes closest to describing yourself.

Please answer *all* questions and work through from first to last without
going back over your answers.

Scoring

For each C: If yes, 0 points
          If no, 1 point

For each S: If yes, 2 points
          If no, 0 points

For each A: If yes, 2 points
          If no, 0 points

For each N: If yes, 2 points
          If no, 0 points

(Please note that C is the exception here, a yes carries 0 points but a
no carries 1 point.)
Total number of points: 91
For interpretation see end of questionnaire.

Code					Points
C	1	I can take a measured look at a job to be done without feeling an urge to rush into action before getting the thing properly sorted out.	YES	NO	0
S	2	I have recently had to give up an important personal relationship	YES	NO	2
N	3	I often need understanding friends to cheer me up.	YES	NO	2
C	4	I can control my temper; when I lose it, this is calculated, I don't go beyond what I intended to say or do.	YES	NO	0
C	5	I find it easy to get along with and accept people who hold different points of view to my own.	YES	NO	0
N	6	My mood often goes up and down	YES	NO	0
A	7	Having to tolerate delays of any kind is very irritating to me.	YES	NO	0
A	8	I prefer to assume complete responsibility rather than sharing it with others.	YES	NO	0
S	9	Recent events in my life have forced an important change in my social relationships.	YES	NO	
A	10	I do not suffer fools gladly.	YES	NO	
C	11	I can focus on one thing when necessary and clear my mind of other things to be done.	YES	NO	
A	12	I take pride in getting the job done faster than most.	YES	NO	
N	13	I sometimes feel 'just miserable' for no good reason.	YES	NO	
N	14	My feelings are rather easily hurt.	YES	NO	
A	15	Deadlines are very important to me.	YES	NO	
C	16	I can say 'no' to people who make an unreasonable demand without them being too upset.	YES	NO	
S	17	My sexual needs are largely unsatisfied.	YES	NO	
C	18	I usually try to deal with problems systematically and in an organised way.	YES	NO	
A	19	I have plenty of battles on my hands at work.	YES	NO	
S	20	I have suffered considerably from constant arguments at home and at work.	YES	NO	
S	21	I have very real financial problems.	YES	NO	
N	22	I am often troubled by feelings of guilt.	YES	NO	
C	23	I can get over disappointments without getting too upset; I recognise that one cannot have everything the way one wishes.	YES	NO	
N	24	I would call myself tense or highly-strung.	YES	NO	
C	25	I can immerse myself in constructive activity as a way of taking my mind away from a problem.	YES	NO	
S	26	I have recently had serious problems in a close relationship.	YES	NO	
C	27	I can usually get other people to see all sides of a problem.	YES	NO	
C	28	I can unwind quickly on a holiday and begin to enjoy myself from the start.	YES	NO	
A	29	I enjoy competing at work and elsewhere.	YES	NO	
C	30	I feel I am as good as the next man.	YES	NO	
C	31	When confronted with a problem I usually remain optimistic about the outcome.	YES	NO	
A	32	I get impatient and angry with incompetence and inefficiency.	YES	NO	
N	33	I get attacks of shaking or trembling.	YES	NO	
A	34	I work long hours from choice.	YES	NO	
S	35	I or members of my family, have recently experienced problems due to illness.	YES	NO	

N	36	I am an irritable person.	YES	NO	☐
A	37	I drive myself harder than most.	YES	NO	☐
C	38	I can usually break down a problem into manageable chunks.	YES	NO	☐
N	39	I worry about awful things that might happen.	YES	NO	☐
N	40	I would call myself a nervous person.	YES	NO	☐
C	41	I can count on the support of my family and friends.	YES	NO	☐
S	42	I have to spend too much time away from home.	YES	NO	☐
A	43	I am very ambitious	YES	NO	☐
N	44	I am easily hurt when people find fault with me or my work.	YES	NO	☐
S	45	I sometimes have to assume responsibility for events over which I have no control.	YES	NO	☐
N	46	I am troubled by feelings of inferiority.	YES	NO	☐
S	47	Someone close to me has recently died.	YES	NO	☐
S	48	At times I have more work than I feel able to cope with.	YES	NO	☐
C	49	I am able to tell other people what I feel and think; I do not simmer privately or explode.	YES	NO	☐
A	50	I tend to get involved in many different ideas and projects.	YES	NO	☐
N	51	I suffer from sleeplessness.	YES	NO	☐
S	52	I have to work with others of unpredictable and uncertain temperament.	YES	NO	☐
S	53	I feel dissatisfied at work due to e.g.: blocked promotion, threat of redundancy, excessive demands of superiors etc.	YES	NO	☐

Total Points _____

Interpretation of score

0 – 24 points

In terms of stress, personality type and coping skills, you are in a low coronary risk category. Whatever life stresses are present you appear to cope quite well and you do not appear to be under any undue pressure.

25 – 50 points

You evidently have some pressure and stress but in general manage to cope. Your levels of stress and tension are acceptable for most of the time and are not generally at levels where it is likely to cause you any harm. Much of your tension and stress is productive and should not, therefore, be viewed negatively.

51 – 70 points

You are now moving into a category of personality type and stress which is more akin to the 'coronary prone' group. Sometimes the stress and tension can make you feel uncomfortable and you may find it difficult to cope adequately. You tend to feel 'stretched' or 'pushed' a lot of the time although you may sometimes find this enjoyable. You are probably prone to fluctuations in mood. With scores at this level you may run the risk of ill-health if the pressure continues unremittingly.

More than 70

This is a high risk category. The levels of tension and stress and therefore inter-action with your personality type, suggest you are 'coronary prone' and perhaps also susceptible to other forms of illness and disease. You may have problems sleeping and your alcohol consumption may have increased. You may be using various forms of tranquillisers and sedativs and have the constant feeling you are unable to cope. Continuing to live at this sort of intensity may well result in eventual break-down, both physical and mental.

Appendix 3

Your Target Heart Rates

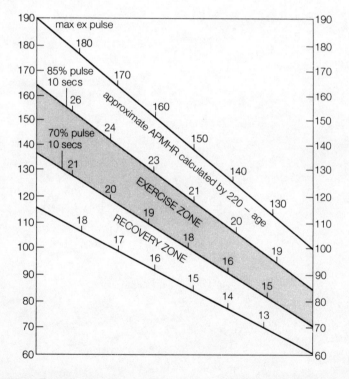

Figure A3.1   Target heart rates.

Figure A3.1 shows a rough way of assessing the suitable intensity of exercise as gauged by heart rate. Calculate your approximate maximum heart rate by subtracting your age from 220. For example, if you are 40 years of age your age predicted maximum heart rate (APMHR) is 180 beats.

You will see that with an APMHR of 180, the appropriate intensity of exercise should be between 21 and 26 beats over a ten-second count. This represents an intensity of 70–85 per cent of your age predicted maximum heart rate.

If you are 60 years old then your APMHR is 160. From the chart you will see that the appropriate heart rate for exercise is between 19 and 23 beats over a ten-second count which again represents 70–85 per cent of your age predicted maximum.

Appendix 4
Flexibility Exercises

These flexibility exercises are an important part of your training programme. Adequate stretching and flexing of muscles prior to exercise can do much to reduce the chances of injury. They take only a few minutes to perform and if you use three or four each week you can vary them according to your wishes.

Lower leg and heel stretcher

Purpose	To stretch the muscles of the lower leg and the Achilles' tendon.
Start	Stand upright approximately 3 feet from a wall or post
Movement	Keeping the feet flat on the floor, extend the arms forward touching the wall and slowly allow the body to lean forward, holding the stretched position for 5 seconds. You will feel the tension in the back of the calves and upper leg.
Repetitions	10 – 15 times or more.
Note	This is a very important exercise prior to running.

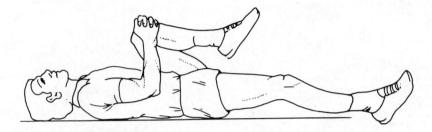

Single knee to chest

Purpose	To stretch muscles in the lower back and buttocks.
Start	Lie on the back with the legs extended forward.
Movement	Bring the right knee up and into the chest, pulling the knee with the hands and arms as far forward as possible, hold in the fully stretched position for 5 seconds, and then repeat with the opposite leg.
Repetitions	10 times or more for each leg.

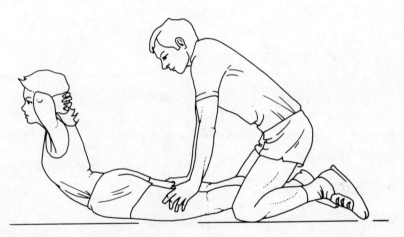

Back hyperextension

Purpose	To stretch the abdominal and chest muscles and to strengthen the lower back.
Start	Lie on the stomach, with the legs extended to the rear, and the hands behind the head.
Movement	With a partner holding the feet, slowly extend the trunk upward as far as possible and hold for 3 to 5 seconds.
Repetitions	10 times or more.
Note	If you do not have a partner then you can hook your feet under a heavy object, for example a piece of furniture.

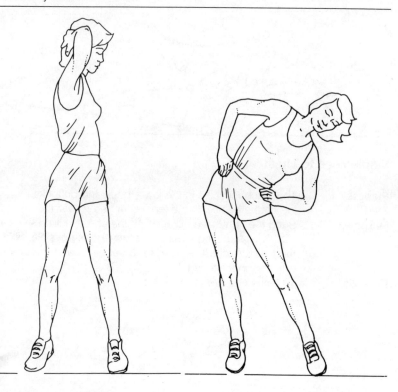

Trunk rotation (*left*)

Purpose	To stretch the muscles of the back, sides, and shoulder girdle.
Start	Stand upright, hands behind the head, and the feet placed shoulder-width apart.
Movement	Rotate the trunk as far to the right as possible, and then rotate as far to the left as possible.
Repetitions	10 times or more to each side.

Hip rotation (*right*)

Purpose	To stretch the muscles of the hips and back.
Start	Stand upright, hands on hips, with the feet placed shoulder-width apart.
Movement	Bending at the waist, rotate the trunk to the right side, forward, left side, and return.
Repetitions	10 times or more.

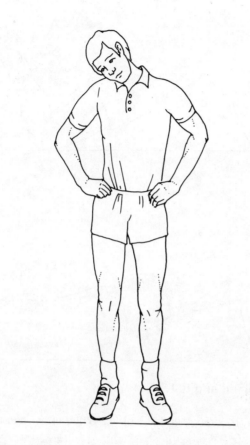

Head rotation

Purpose	To stretch the muscles of the neck and upper back.
Start	Standing upright with the hands on the hips, and the feet placed shoulder-width apart.
Movement	Slowly rotate the head clockwise in a full circle for the specified number of repetitions; then reverse the direction for an equal number of repetitions.
Repetitions	Repeat 10 times or more.
Note	Perform this exercise *gently*.

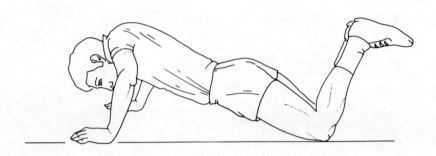

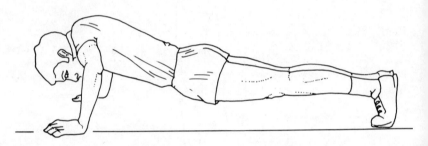

Push-up, modified and full

Purpose	To strengthen the muscles of the upper arm and shoulder girdle.
Start	Arms fully extended, shoulder-width apart supporting the upper body weight, with the feet extended backward, the toes supporting the lower body weight.
Movement	Slowly lower the chest to the floor, keeping the back straight and in line with the buttocks, then push back up to the fully extended position.
Repetitions	10 times or more.
Note	For those with limited upper body strength, perform this exercise with the knees on the floor, forming the point of support. Move to the full push-up when 30 repetitions can be performed.

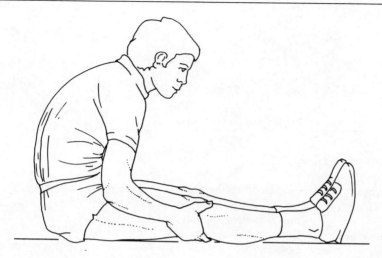

Pike position

Purpose   To stretch the hamstrings and lower back muscles.
Start   Assume a sitting position with the legs extended forward
               and the knees pressed flat on the floor.
Movement   Grasp behind the knees and slowly pull the trunk down
               towards the knees, holding the stretched position for 5
               seconds.
Repetitions   10 times or more.

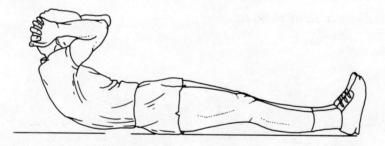

Head and shoulder curl

Purpose   To stretch the muscles of the neck and upper back and to
               promote abdominal strength.
Start   Lie on the back with the legs fully extended forward and the
               hands behind the head or neck.
Movement   Slowly curl the head and shoulders forward to approximately
               a 45° position, and hold for 5 seconds.
Repetitions   10 – 15 times or more

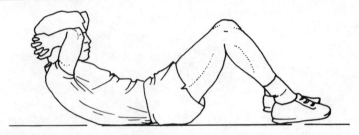

Bent-knee sit-up

Purpose   To strengthen the abdominal and hip flexor muscles.
Start   Lie on the back with the knees bent to a 90° angle, and the hands clasped behind the head.
Movement   Curl the head, shoulders and back up to the full sitting position touching one of the knees with the opposite elbow.
Repetitions 10 times or more
Note   If you find the exercise difficult to perform with the knees bent, then you can start with the knees straight.

Glossary of Terms

Aerobic: Exercise that is dependent upon oxygen.

Anaerobic: Exercise that is non-oxygen-dependent. Because of this and because it results in the accumulation of waste products, e.g. lactic acid, it can only take place for short periods of time. Examples of anaerobic activity are sprinting and weight training etc. where short, explosive bursts of power are required.

Angina: Chest pain, usually due to coronary artery disease.

Arteriosclerosis: Literally, 'Hardening of the arteries'. A general term that refers to the progressive narrowing and hardening of the arteries which accompanies the ageing process.

Atherogenic: Promoting the formation of atheroma, e.g. an atherogenic diet is one which encourages the deposition of fat in the arterial wall.

Atheroma: The 'furring up' of the arteries with progressive narrowing of the artery.

Atherosclerosis: For practical purposes, this is the same as arterio-sclerosis.

Carbohydrate: A chemical compound consisting of carbon, hydrogen and oxygen atoms in specified arrangements. Carbohydrates are measured components of foods such as bread, potatoes and rice.

Cardiac: Pertaining to the heart.

Cardiac output: The volume of blood pumped from the heart per unit of time. Each time the heart contracts a volume of blood is ejected into the circulation. This volume of blood is called the stroke volume. When this is multiplied by the heart rate (i.e. beats per minute) the result obtained is termed cardiac output: e.g. if the heart rate is 65 beats per minute and if the stroke volume (the amount ejected per beat) is 77 ml (millilitres), then the cardiac output is $77 \times 65 = 5$ litres. During vigorous exercise the heart rate may increase to 195 beats per minute and the stroke volume increased to 154 ml, giving a cardiac output of $195 \times 154 = 30$ litres.

Cardiovascular: Pertaining to the heart and the arteries.

Cholesterol: An important component of the blood fats (lipids) which has been strongly associated with heart disease. It is essential to understand, however, that it also has a vital role in the normal functioning of the body. It is found only in animal products. Levels of cholesterol in the blood are measured in millimoles per litre (mmol/l).

Coronary angiography: A special technique whereby a special dye is injected into the coronary arteries and a sophisticated camera is used to take a series of pictures. The technique allows direct visualization of the arteries and is always performed prior to coronary artery surgery.

Coronary atheroma: Atheroma (i.e. 'furring up' of the arteries) occurring in the coronary artery system.

Coronary bypass surgery: Also referred to as coronary artery bypass grafting (CABG). In this operation, veins are removed from the legs and are used to bypass narowed or blocked coronary arteries.

Coronary heart disease: The narrowing which occurs in the coronary arteries and which usually produces symptoms such as angina or heart attacks.

Coronary thrombosis: A heart attack. Often referred to as simply a 'coronary'.

Diabetes: The condition in which insulin is either deficient or defective and the level of the blood sugar rises.

Diastole: (Diastolic) The resting phase of the heart. The diastolic blood pressure is the pressure in the arterial system, whilst the heart is at rest. It is the lower of the two blood pressures.

Electrocardiograph: (ECG) An electrical record of the activity of the heart muscle. The process of making these records is electrocardiography.

Epidemiology: The study of disease patterns within populations.

False-Negative: A term used in exercise stress testing. It is when the study of an ECG during exercise is normal although the individual does in fact have heart disease. In other words, the test has failed to identify the disease.

False-Positive: A term used in exercise stress testing. It is a situation in which the exercise ECG is abnormal, even though the individual does not have heart disease. In other words, the ECG suggests that he does have disease when in fact he is normal.

Fitness: The capacity to perform work.

Genetic: An in-built or constitutional predisposition: e.g. in coronary heart disease some individuals have a predisposition which is handed on to them by their parents.

Glycogen: Made up of glucose molecules, it is the storage form of carbohydrate in the muscle.

Hyperlipidaemia: Also termed hyperlipoproteinaemia. Conditions in which the blood lipids (fats) are increased. Raised blood cholesterol is one of the most important forms of hyperlipidaemia.

Hypertension: Raised blood pressure.

Incidence: The incidence of a disease is the number of new cases of the disease occurring annually.

Lipids: The blood fats.

Maximum oxygen consumption: ($\dot{V}O_2$ max) The greatest volume of oxygen which is used by the muscles per unit of time. It is a measure of cardiorespiratory fitness.

Metabolism: The sum total of physiological and biochemical reaction within the body, which provides energy for movement and materials for the repair and growth of the organism.

MET capacity: An expression of the energy cost relative to each individual's resting energy expenditure. 1 MET equals the energy used at rest. Therefore, 10 MET is ten times the energy required to support the body at rest. As an example, a hard game of squash would require 15 to 17 METs, whereas most gardening activities require only 5 to 7 METs.

Morbidity: Disability caused by disease.

Mortality: The mortality rate is the number of deaths within a community from a given disease. It is usually expressed per 100,000 of the population.

Myocardial infarction: Heart attack.

Myocardium: Heart muscle.

Obesity: Excess body fat.

Overweight: Excess body fat, but not sufficiently excessive to be termed obese.

Prevalence: The prevalence of disease is the amount of disease within a population at any given time.

Readiness for living: Can be defined precisely as the difference between the available physical energy an individual has to complete a task and the fatigue imposed upon that individual at the time of performing that specific task.

Resting heart rate: The heart rate at rest can vary in healthy individuals from as low as 40 beats per minute (in the athletically trained) to 80 beats per minute. It can also vary at different times during the day and tends to be at its lowest during sleep.

Sedentary: Inactive

Stress testing: Usually refers to exercise stress testing. A sophisticated technique of following the function of the heart by taping electrodes to the chest wall and observing the electrocardiograph during created exercise.

Stroke: A brain haemorrhage.

Stroke Volume: The amount of blood ejected from the heart during each contraction.

Systole: (Systolic) The active contraction of the heart. The systolic blood pressure is, therefore, the arterial pressure during that contraction phase.

Triglycerides: Another type of fat found in the blood, large quantities of which are associated with heart disease. The association, however, is not as strong as that between cholesterol and heart disease.

List of Major Works Cited

Amery A., Bulpitt C. et al., 'Does diet matter in hypertension?' *European Heart Journal* (forthcoming).

Bassler T. J., 1972. 'Athletic Activity and Longevity', *Lancet*, 2: 712.

Bassler T. J., 1973. 'Long Distance Runners', *Science*, 182: 113.

Bassler T. J., Cardello F. P., 1976. 'Fiber Feeding and Atherosclerosis', *Journal of the American Medical Association*, 235: 1841–2.

Brunner D., Manelis G., 1960. 'Myocardial Infarction among Members of Communal Settlements in Israel', *Lancet* 2: 1049.

Chapman J. M., Goerke L. S. et al., 1957. 'The Clinical Status of a Population Group in Los Angeles under Observation for Two to Three Years', *American Journal of Public Health*, 47, supplement: 33–42.

Committee on Medical Aspects of Food Policy (COMA), 1984. Report of the Panel on Diet in Relation to Cardio-vascular disease (Dept of Health and Social Security Report on Health and Social Subjects 28).

Cooper K. H., Pollock M. L. et al., 1976. 'Physical Fitness Levels vs. Selected Coronary Risk Factors', *Journal of the American Medical Association*, 236: 166–9.

Eckstein R. W., 1957. 'Effect of Exercise and Coronary Artery Narrowing on Coronary Collateral Circulation', *Circulation Research*, 5: 230–5.

Friedman M. and Roseman R. H., 1959. *Journal of the American Medical Association*, 169: 1286.

Garcia-Palmieri M. R., Costas R. et al., 1982. 'Increased Physical Activity: a Protective Factor against Heart Attacks in Puerto Rico', *American Journal of Cardiology*, 50, 749–55.

Hames C. D., 1971. 'Evans County Cardiovascular and Cerebrovascular Epidemiologic Study', *Archives of Internal Medicine*, 128 (6).

Hellerstein, H. K., Boyer J. L., 1976. 'Exploring the Effects of Exercise on Hypertension', *Physician Sportsmed* 4 (12): 36–49.

Kahn H. A., 1963. 'The Relationship of Reported Coronary Heart Disease Mortality to Physical Activity of Work', *American Journal of Public Health*, 53: 1058.

Kannel W. B., Gordon T., 1970. *The Framingham Study*, Sections 24, 26. Washington, DC: US Government Printing Office.

Keys A., ed., 1970. 'Summary: Coronary Heart Disease in Seven Countries', *Circulation*, 41–2, supplement I: 186–95.

Kramsch D. et al., 1981. 'Reduction of Coronary Atherosclerosis by Moderate Conditioning Exercise in Monkeys on an Atherogenic Diet', *New England Journal of Medicine*, 305 (25), 1483–9.

Lipid Research Clinics Program, 1984. The Lipid Research Clinics Coronary Primary Prevention Trial Results: 1, 'Reduction in Incidence of Coronary Hearth Disease', and 2, 'The Relationship of Reduction in Incidence of Coronary Heart Disease to Cholesterol Lowering', *Journal of American Medical Association*, 251: 351–64, 365–74.

McDonough J. R., Hames C. G., Stolb S. C., Garrison G. E., 1965. 'Coronary Heart Disease among Negroes and Whites in Evans County, Georgia', *Journal of Chronic Disease*, 18: 443–68.

Malhotra S. L., 1967. 'Epidemiology of Ischaemic Heart Disease in India with Special Reference to Causation', *British Heart Journal*, 29: 895.

Morris J. N., Adam C. et al., 1973. 'Vigorous Exercise in Leisure-Time and the Incidence of Coronary Heart Disease', *Lancet*, i, 333–9.

Morris J. N., Pollard R. et al., 1980. 'Vigorous Exercise in Leisure-Time: Protection against Coronary Heart Disease', *Lancet*, ii, 1207–10.

National Advisory Committee on Nutrition Education (NACNE), 1983. 'A discussion paper on proposals for nutritional guidance for health education in Britain', prepared for NACNE by an ad hoc working party under the Chairmanship of Professor W. P. T. James. Health Education Council Document.

Noakes T. D., Opie L. H., 1979. 'Marathon Running and Heart: the South African Experience', *American Heart Journal* 98; 669–71.

Noakes T. D., Opie L. H. et al., 1979. 'Autopsy Proven Coronary Atherosclerosis in Marathon Runners', *New England Journal of Medicine* 301: 86–89.

Northcote R. J., MacFarlane P., Ballantyne D,. 1983. 'Ambulatory Electrocardiography in Squash Players', *British Heart Journal* 50 (4): 372–7.

Northcote R. J., Evans A. D., Ballantyne D., 1984. 'Sudden Death in Squash Players', *Lancet*, i, 8369: 148–50.

Opie L. H., 1975. 'Sudden Death and Sport', *Lancet*, 263–6.

Paffenbarger R. S., Hale W. E., 1975. 'Work Activity and Coronary Heart Mortality', *New England Journal of Medicine*, 292 (11).

Paffenbarger R. S., Wing A. L., Hyde R. T., 1967. 'Physical Activity as an Index of Heart Attack Risk in College Alumni', *American Journal of Epidemiology*, 108: 161.

Pomrehn, P. R., Wallace R. B., Burmeister L. F., 1982. 'Ischaemic Heart Disease Mortality in Iowa Farmers', *Journal of the American Medical Association*, 248 (9).

Rosenman R. H., Brand R. J., Scholtz R. I., Friedman M., 1976. *American Journal of Cardiology* 37: 903–9.

Shapiro S., Weinblatt E. et al., 1969. 'Incidence of Coronary Heart Disease in a Population Insured for Medical Care (HIP)', *American Journal of Public Health*, 59, supplement II, (6) 1–101.

Shephard R. J., 1974. 'Sudden Death – a Significant Hazard of Exercise', *British Journal of Sports Medicine*, 8: 101–10.

Solomons H. 1984. 'The Exercise Myth'. Angus & Robertson.

Stamler J., Farinaro E. et al. 1980. 'Prevention and Control of Hypertension by Nutritional-hygienic means', *Journal of the American Medical Association* 243: 1819–23.

Stamler J., Lindberg H. A., et al. 1960. 'Prevalence and Incidence of Coronary Heart Disease in Strata of the Labor Force of a Chicago Industrial Corporation', *Journal of Chronic Disease*: 11 (4) 405–20.

Stone M. C., Thorp J. M., 1984. 'Plasma fibrinogen – a major coronary risk factor', in Lenzi S., Descoich G. C., eds, *Atherosclerosis and Cardiovascular Disease*: 3–10. Bologna, Editric Compositors.

Taylor M. L., Klepetar E. et al. 1962. 'Death Rates among Physically Active and Sedentary Employees of the Railroad Industry', *American Journal of Public Health*, 52: 2967.

Thompson P. D., Funk E. J. et al. 1982. 'Incidence of Death During Jogging in Rhode Island from 1975 through 1980', *Journal of the American Medical Association* 247: 2535–8.

Waller B. F., Roberts W. C., 1980. 'Sudden Death while Running in Conditioned Runners aged 40 Years or Over', *American Journal of Cardiology*, 45: 1295–1300.

Zukel W. J., Lewis W. J. et al., 1959. 'A Short-term Community Study of the Epidemiology of Coronary Heart Disease', *American Journal of Public Health*, 49: 1630.

Index